Rosemary

The Healing Herb of St. Martin de Porres

By Charles S. Brocato (Dr. "B")

Cover Photo: istock.com/Creativeeye99

Back Cover: istock.com/LukeLuke68

All Other Photos: Charles S. Brocato

Dedicated to my mother, Jhovita E. Brocato

Table of Contents

Introduction

Charles S. Brocato, known to his students as Dr. "B," became fascinated with the herb known as rosemary when he studied the life of St. Martin de Porres, who lived in Lima, Peru, just after the Conquistadors had conquered the area and established Lima as the new capital city.

Martin de Porres was born the son of a Spanish knight and a free black woman in 1579. He trained as a barber when barbers not only gave haircuts, but also treated wounds and sicknesses. Martin developed above-average skills.

Soon afterward, at the age of 15, he entered the Holy Rosary Priory in Lima and became a Dominican *donado*, acting as a servant in the convent. His exceptional holiness was recognized by the prior, and at the age of 24, he professed religious vows.

He was assigned to the infirmary, where his skills combined with his friendship with God. He became known all over Lima for his care of the sick and for the miracles of healing he often performed. He never distinguished between persons of high rank or low when he treated his patients. Even sick or injured animals knew to come to St. Martin for treatment.

St. Martin's favorite remedies often involved rosemary, whether as a fragrant branch burned as an air purifier or as an extract in wine that he used to clean wounds. Although the saint probably did not need physical means to effect his cures (a glass of plain water given by St. Martin healed sicknesses), he always employed them when he could, and he often put rosemary to good use.

Upon researching the herb, Dr. "B" found that rosemary, like many spices, has a myriad of uses and probably even more effects on the body, but because it cannot be patented, we may never know just how powerful rosemary is and all the ailments it might be good for. There is no money in it, so drug companies will not sponsor research that isn't likely to yield a patentable drug.

However, research is taking place around the world, and much of what has been done strongly suggests every home needs a rosemary bush or two in a sunny spot of the garden or in a place of honor in a flowerbed.

Dr. "B" believes almost anyone can benefit from rosemary, the healing herb favored by St. Martin de Porres.

1: What Is Rosemary?

Most of us are familiar with rosemary as a spice that looks like chopped-up pine needles, with a delicious smell that goes really well when cooked into meat-based dishes.

Indeed, rosemary, scientifically known as *Rosmarinus officinalis*, is a traditional spice of long standing that is native to the Mediterranean region. It is grouped by botanists into the Laminaceae or mint family, which includes other herbs such as marjoram, oregano, peppermint, spear-mint, sage and thyme.

According to the online encyclopedia, Wikipedia, the name rosemary comes from the Latin words for dew (*ros*) and sea (*marinus*), or *dew of the sea*. It tends to flower constantly in warm climates, with flowers of white, pink, purple, or deep blue. Legend says that the Virgin Mary rested beside a rosemary bush and spread her blue cloak over it. The white flowers turned blue, and the herb was called the "Rose of Mary."

Rosemary is an evergreen shrub that thrives in many North American gardens, especially in the more southern regions. Like many mints, it may help repel pests from other garden plants.

Its aromatic leaves are used in cooking, as it has anti-bacterial effects on foods and lends a delightful flavor to many dishes, such as stuffings and meats. The use of spices in cooking is believed to have originated because (1) they added excellent flavor to otherwise bland foods, and (2) they helped retard spoilage of the food.

Rosemary has a long history of use in cosmetic preparations. Hungary water, first made for Elisabeth of Poland, Queen of Hungary, was made by soaking the tips of rosemary plants in wine. Current recipes include rosemary in addition to many other aromatic herbs. Hungary water is considered one of the first perfumes.

Because of the highly fragrant oils rosemary contains, it has a long history of usage in incenses and in cosmetic preparations, not to mention perfumes.

Remembrance

Ophelia, in Shakespeare's *Hamlet*, says, "There's rosemary, that's for remembrance." Since *Hamlet* was written around the year 1600, we can surmise rosemary had been associated with remembrance a long time before that.

Because of this association with remembrance, rosemary signifies just that in war ceremonies and funerals in Europe and Australia. In Australia, people wear sprigs of rosemary on ANZAC Day to commemorate the landing of Australian and New Zealand troops in Gallipolli, Turkey, in World War I, and often on Remembrance Day, November 1, when all the war dead are remembered.

Rosemary also has a long history of use for improving the memory. Wikipedia notes a report from *The Guardian* that in 2017, rosemary oil sales to UK students preparing for exams had "skyrocketed, because of rosemary's perceived benefits to memory."

This is believable because peppermint, another member of the mint family, has this same property. Studies have shown that if students breathe in the peppermint fragrance, their memories are sharper and they retain more of what they study.

Medical Uses

Traditionally, Rosemary was used in medicine to treat a variety of disorders, and considering the many chemicals the herb contains that are known to have medicinal benefits, this is hardly surprising.

As we have noted, St. Martin de Porres favored rosemary greatly, and one of his most trusted remedies was wine that had been heated with rosemary.

According to *St. Martin de Porres: Apostle of Charity*:

> Martin took him (an injured dog) by the ear and led him off to his own room, where he washed the wounds with wine in which rosemary had been heated – one of his infallible remedies – and then began to sew them up.

In the days of St. Martin, a sickroom was probably a stuffy and possibly odiferous place. St. Martin used rosemary twigs to sweeten the air.

> Martin often passed through locked doors, carrying voluminous objects with him, such as sheets and other linens, or his famous brazier, filled with burning coals. He would suddenly appear to a sick member of the community in the middle of the night. Placing the brazier on the floor, he would throw a branch of rosemary on the coals, and at once the cheerful crackling and delightful perfume of the rosemary dispelled the heaviness of the vitiated air in the cell.

How Rosemary Is Used Today

Rosemary is used today in four major ways:

1. As a *spice*, to add flavor to food and to help preserve it against spoilage.

2. As an *herb*, in the form of capsules and tea, for medicinal purposes

3. As an *essential oil*, used in cosmetics, shampoos and other items for the body.

4. As an alcohol *extract*, for use on the skin or to take internally.

We believe rosemary will still do all the things Martin de Porres used it for then; today, and very likely more. Let us first examine just what is in this marvelous plant that makes it so beneficial.

2: *What Does Rosemary Contain?*

Rosemary is known to contain several important *phyto-chemicals*, or chemicals contained in plants

In alphabetic order, rosemary contains the following phyto-chemicals:

Alpha-pinene: An organic chemical of the terpene class (organic, aromatic chemicals produced by plants such as conifers) that is found in many coniferous trees, such as pine trees. It is anti-inflammatory, helps improve breathing, helps short-term memory loss and promotes alertness.

Apigenin: A flavone (a basis of white or yellow plant pigments) found in many plants that may have many beneficial effects in humans, although little research has been done in people. It may prevent renal damage and stimulate adult neurogenesis, or rebuilding or nerves. It may also prevent the beta amyloid deposition characteristic of Alzheimer's disease. It has also been shown effective against many cancer types, without toxicity to normal cells.

Beta-carotene: A red-orange pigment of the carotenoid class found in carrots and other yellow/orange vegetables. It is a precursor to Vitamin A and is a known antioxidant.

Beta sitosterol: A well-known *phytosterol* (plant sterol) that is believed to help reduce benign prostatic hyperplasia and blood cholesterol levels.

Betulinic acid: A triterpenoid (a subclass of the terpenes) that occurs in many tree barks. It is known to have anti-inflammatory, antimalarial and antiretroviral properties, besides showing potential as an anticancer agent.

Borneol: An organic terpene derivative that occurs naturally in some plants like camphorweed, wormwood and sagebrush. It has antibacterial and analgesic (pain-relieving) properties and is used to help relieve the pain and itching of hemorrhoids. It is a part of many Chinese herbal remedies and is said to help prevent cardiovascular disease, aid the digestive system, treat bronchitis and to promote relaxation.

Caffeic acid: An organic compound found in all plants, as it is a key intermediate in the formation of lignin. It is classified as a hydroxycinnamic acid and is found in many spices like sage, spearmint and thyme, Ceylon cinnamon and star anise. It is also found in red wine, yerba mate and black chokeberry, among other foods. Caffeic acid is an anti-inflammatory, a natural fungicide and has been shown to inhibit cancer cell proliferation.

Camphor: Classified as a terpenoid (known for aromatic qualities) found in the camphor laurel, and in amounts of 10 to 20% in rosemary. Camphor is antimicrobial and repels insects. It has long been used for its decongestant effects and is a chief ingredient in Vicks VapoRub.

Carvacrol: Classified as a monoterpenoid, carvacrol is responsible for the odor of oregano oil. The essential oils of thyme, wild bergamot and marjoram also contain carvacrol. It inhibits the growth of several strains of bacteria, notably *Escherichia coli*, *Bacillus cerus*, and *Pseudomonas aeruginosa*, all of which are involved in food spoilage and food poisoning. Besides its known antibacterial actions, carvacrol may have anticancer effects.

Carvone: A terpene that is found in many essential oils, notably caraway, dill and spearmint. It is used commercially in foods like spearmint-flavored candies and gums, and to stop premature sprouting of potatoes. It also has insect-repelling qualities.

Carophyllene: Belongs to a subclass of the terpenes, and is a constituent of many essential oils, notably cannabis, cloves, hops and rosemary. It has anti-inflammatory actions and is neuroprotective, antibacterial, antifungal and anticancer.

Chlorogenic acid: An ester of caffeic acid that occurs naturally in many plants, like bamboo and heather. An isomer occurs in coffee. It has been shown to help reduce blood pressure and possibly has anti-inflammatory effects.

Diosmin: A flavone that is found particularly in a plant of the Iberian Penninsula, *Teucrium gnaphalodes*. It is used in treating spider and varicose veins, and has anti-inflammatory and blood-sugar-lowering effects.

Genkwanin: A flavone that is found in seeds of the common alder tree and certain ferns. It appears to have anti-inflammatory and antitumor effects.

Geraniol: A monoterpene and an alcohol that is the primary constituent of rose oil, palmarosa oil and citronella oil, and occurs in smaller amounts in many other oils. It is used commercially in flavors such as blueberry, grapefruit, lemon, peach, raspberry and pineapple. It has antioxidant and anti-inflammatory properties, and has potent antitumor and anti-cancer effects.

Hesperidin: A compound found in citrus peels and in peppermint. It is a precursor to the flavonoid herperitin, which helps increase circulation and possibly has brain-protective effects.

Limonene: A terpene found in mint oils and citrus peels that has a pine-like odor. It appears to have anticancer properties and is used to treat bronchitis. It is also used as a flavoring agent in foods and beverages.

Linalool: A terpene alcohol found in many spices and flowers. Over 200 species of plants produce linalool, including the members of the mint family. It is used in many personal hygiene products and cleaning agents, and as an insecticide for fleas and cockroaches.

Luteolin: A flavone most often found in leaves, such as oregano, parsley, thyme, rosemary and peppermint. It is an antioxidant with anti-inflammatory and anticancer effects, and may have a role in cancer prevention.

Oleanolic acid: Another member of the terpene family that is found in olive oil, pokeweed, juniper mistletoe and honey mesquite. It helps protect the liver and has anticancer and antiviral properties.

1,8-cineole: A terpene known more popularly as eucalyptol as it comprises 90% of the essential oil of eucalyptus oil. Because of its scent and flavor, it is used in many cosmetics and food products. It also has insect killing and repelling qualities. It helps relieve symptoms of bronchitis and has anti-inflammatory properties.

Phytosterols: Structurally similar to cholesterol, but produced by plants. When consumed, they compete with cholesterol for absorption and thus have cholesterol-lowering effects. Beta sitosterol is one of the major phytosterols.

Rosmanol: An antioxidant and antibacterial compound found in rosemary and sage.

Rosmarinic acid: An ester (a compound formed by reacting a carboxylic acid with an alcohol) found in many culinary herbs like basil, holy basil, lemon balm, marjoram, peppermint, rosemary, sage and thyme, and in other plant species. It is considered a potential anti-anxiety treatment, plus it has antiviral effects and is used against Herpes simplex virus type-2. It also has anti-inflammatory activity and strong anti-oxidant properties.

Salicylates: Salts or esters of salicylic acid that are found in many plants and food plants like white willow bark and wintergreen leaves. They are known, like aspirin, for their powerful anti-inflammatory effects.

Squalene: A triterpene derived commercially from shark liver oil, but also found in plants like aramanth seed, rice bran, wheat germ and olives. It is a precursor for synthesis of plant and animal sterols, including cholesterol and steroid hormones in the human body.

Tannin: A polyphenol (an organic chemical containing multiple phenol units) that is widely distributed among plants, probably to help prevent animals from eating the plant. It is famous for its use in treating leathers. It also has antibacterial qualities, particularly against foodborne bacteria.

Thymol: A member of the terpene family that is found in thyme oil and is considered an isomer (same chemical formula) of carvacrol. It has antimicrobial, antifungal and relaxing qualities

Ursolic acid: A member of the terpene family of chemicals that is found in the peelings of fruits, particularly in apple peelings, as well as in herbs like rosemary and thyme. It appears to have anticancer effects, as well as nerve regenerative properties. In the bodybuilding world, it is known for supposedly supporting lean muscle and helping with fat loss.

Many of these chemicals occur in miniscule amounts, especially considering that people do not use large amounts of rosemary in the first place.

But some of these chemicals are quite powerful and do not need to occur in large amounts in order to confer their effects to the body.

Vitamin & Mineral Content

Rosemary contains quite a few nutrients, and how much it contributes to your daily intake of nutrients naturally depends upon how much rosemary you ingest in a day.

The herb contains a number of B vitamins, including folic acid, pantothenic acid, pyridoxine (B-6) and riboflavin (B-2). It also contains Vitamin C and beta carotene, which the body can convert into Vitamin A if you are not diabetic.

Many herbal references claim that rosemary contains Vitamin A. It does not. Only animal-source foods like liver or butter contain real Vitamin A. Beta-carotene is properly called "pro" Vitamin A, because your body can convert it into real Vitamin A. As noted above, diabetics do not tend to convert beta-carotene into Vitamin A.

As for minerals, rosemary contains calcium, copper, iron, magnesium and manganese.

Judging from its contents, we can see why Martin de Porres got so much use from rosemary, and we believe it is even more useful today than we imagine. For a closer look at the many nutrients in rosemary, go here:

http://nutritiondata.self.com/facts/spices-and-herbs/206/2

In this book we will examine some of the medicinal purposes rosemary is used for, both today and in past times.

3: *Rosemary for the Heart & Nerves*

Rosemary has traditionally been used to boost the blood circulation, especially in older people who may have chronic poor circulation. It is termed a "cardio tonic," meaning it tones up the heart muscles and improves heart function. Exactly how it works is a matter of pharmacological debate.

The herbal extract appears to stimulate smooth muscle activity, besides helping against pain. The diosmin in rosemary is known to reduce capillary fragility and permeability, which makes it helpful against varicose and spider veins.

Rosemary stimulates the central nervous system and the circulation, which helps low blood pressure. This action on the central nervous system may be due to rosmarinic acid's strong anti-oxidant capabilities.

Rosemary essential oil is said to help tone the circulatory system and to increase circulation when used in massage oil blends.

Heart disease risk factors include high cholesterol, high blood pressure and diabetes, all of which rosemary works against.

With its content of beta sitosterol and other plant sterols, it helps to lower cholesterol.

With its cardio tonic action, it helps to normalize blood pressure by strengthening the heart muscle.

And it contains several flavonoids that inhibit DPP-IV (dipeptidyl peptidase IV), which is the same thing some of the newer diabetes drugs do.

In 2014, a study published in the *Journal of Agricultural and Food Chemistry* by Elvira Gonzalez de Mejia and her colleagues at the Human Nutrition University of Illinois at Urbana-Champaign, gave the results of their investigation into whether or not herbs might be a natural method of lowering blood sugar for people with diabetes who cannot afford expensive medications and find it difficult to adhere to lifestyle changes.

The researchers tested four herbs, using either greenhouse-grown versions or dried commercial herbs and checked for their ability to inhibit the diabetes-related enzyme DPP-IV, and lower the risk of type-2 diabetes. They found, not surprisingly, that Greek oregano and Mexican oregano and rosemary did a better job of inhibiting the enzyme than did the same herbs grown in a greenhouse.

Oddly enough, although the fresh herbs from the greenhouse had the most polyphenols and flavonoids, the commercial spices were better inhibitors of the DPP-IV enzyme.

Of course, the researchers point out that more studies are required to understand how these herbs can play a role in lowering the risk of type-2 diabetes in people before a treatment with the spices can be formulated. But since diabetes is a major risk factor for heart disease, and diabetes has assumed epidemic proportions in the United States, this future treatment likely has a huge potential for a lot more than diabetes.

In May of 2017, researchers writing in the journal *PLOS One* found that rosemary leaves "attenuated cardiac remodeling by improving energy metabolism and decreasing oxidative stress" in rats after cardiac infarction. They say that "rosemary supplementation of 0.02% improved diastolic function and reduced hypertrophy after MI." For rats, they say the equivalent of the rosemary dose of 0.02% and 0.2% would be, for humans, equivalent to 11 mg and 110 mg, respectively.

This means that after suffering a heart attack, rosemary supplementation helped the heart rebuild and rearrange its tissues while also reducing free radical damage and reducing thickening of the heart, and improving heart function.

The Nervous System

Rosemary helps keep the nervous system healthy by combating stress and improving the memory. And indeed, the herb contains powerful anti-oxidants that fight against free-radical damage in the brain.

Rosemary oil, says Daniel Mowrey, in *Proven Herbal Blends: A Rational Approach to Prevention and Remedy*, "calms and soothes irritated nerves and upset stomach, and extinguishes strenuous anxiety."

Furthermore, "The oil contributes substantially to the calming and soothing of tense nerves and muscles."

Because of its stimulating effects on the circulation and central nervous system, it may help "sluggishness" by perking a person up.

Much of rosemary's effects on the nerves may be due to its ability to increase free-radical scavenging, thus preventing oxidative stress and the subsequent rise of the stress hormone, cortisol.

One group of researchers from Italy and Iran observed that rosemary is a rich source of "active antioxidant constituents" that are well absorbed through the gastrointestinal tract and the skin. Moreover, it has neuroprotective effects "in different models of neuroinflammation, neurodegeneration, as well as chemical-induced neurotoxicity and oxidative stress."

This basically means that rosemary can definitely "calm" the nerves and protect them from damage.

A study published in Psychiatry Research investigated the effects of just smelling lavender and rosemary oils. The researchers say that both lavender and rosemary aromas decreased saliva cortisol levels and increased free radical scavenging activity in 22 healthy volunteers. They conclude, "These findings clarify that lavender and rosemary enhance FRSA (free radical scavenging activity) and decrease the stress hormone, cortisol, which protects the body from oxidative stress."

Another study, published in the journal *Holistic Nursing Practice* in 2009, looked at the effects of lavender and rosemary oil on test-taking anxiety among nursing students. They found that "the use of lavender and rosemary essential oil sachets reduced test-taking stress in graduate nursing students as evidenced by lower scores on test anxiety measure, personal statements, and pulse rates."

Scientists in Thailand investigated the effects of inhaling rosemary oil on subjects' feelings, as well as its effects on several physiological indicators of the nervous system. They found that the subjects became more active and claimed they felt "fresher," after inhaling the oil.

Moreover, physiological effects were seen that included significant increases in blood pressure, heart rate and respiratory rate. They concluded that their results "confirm the stimulatory effects of rosemary oil and provide supporting evidence that brainwave activity, autonomic nervous system activity, as well as mood states were all affected by the inhalation of rosemary oil.

From this, we can see that St. Martin de Porres knew what he was doing when he burned those rosemary branches on his brazier. The very odor of the rosemary itself helped his patients begin the healing process.

4: *Rosemary for the Memory & Eyesight*

As we noted earlier, rosemary has long been associated with remembrance and is held to improve concentration and the memory. In ancient Greece, students braided sprigs of rosemary into their hair to help their recall during exams.

Probably because of this long history of rosemary aiding memory, scientists today are still investigating it, and they are finding that rosemary does indeed have positive effects on the memory.

In 2003, scientists published a study on how the odors of rosemary and lavender essential oils affect mood and thinking in healthy adults. They designed the study to see how smelling the essential oils of lavender and rosemary affected "on cognitive performance and mood in healthy volunteers." Subjects performed a computerized cognitive assessment battery in a cubicle containing either one of the two aromas or no odor, and completed mood questionnaires before the odor and after completing the test battery. The researchers found that both essential oils produced measurable effects on cognitive performance, as well as "subjective effects on mood."

Reducing Cognitive Decline in the Elderly

In 2011, scientists decided to investigate the traditional reputation of rosemary for memory by seeing if it might possibly help in "reducing widespread cognitive decline in the elderly." They designed a study that was placebo-controlled and double-blinded, using dried rosemary leaf powder in several dosages then measured speed of memory after administering doses of placebo and rosemary. They discovered that the lowest dose of rosemary powder had a "statistically significant beneficial effect compared with placebo." However, the highest dose (6,000 mg) had "a significant impairing effect." They concluded that, "The positive effect of the dose nearest normal culinary consumption" shows that further work on the effects of low-dose rosemary over a longer term would likely prove very valuable.

Researchers in Spain, using aged rats, set out to prove rosemary extract would enhance the elderly rats' antioxidant status and antioxidant defenses. They found that the extract did this by decreasing several known markers for oxidative stress, and concluded that rosemary extract did indeed improve "the oxidative stress status in old rats." Oxidative stress is known to impair the memory.

Since oxidative stress and free radicals in excess are believed to be a major cause of degeneration and aging, compounds which decrease these are what we call *anti-aging* substances.

A group of Iranian scientists in 2015 investigated the effect of rosemary on spatial memory, learning and "antioxidant enzymes activities in the hippocampus of middle-aged rats." The researchers fed 32 middle-aged male Wistar rats different doses of rosemary extract that was standardized to contain 40% carnosic acid, or distilled water for 12 weeks. They concluded that, "The results revealed that rosemary extract (40% carnosic acid) may improve the memory score and oxidative stress activity in middle-aged rats in a dose dependent manner, especially in 100 mg/kg," which was the medium dose given.

Mild Traumatic Brain Injury

In 2016, researchers looked into whether rosemary extract would improve cognitive deficits in repetitive mild Traumatic Brain Injury (rmTBI) in rats, and possibly how it worked. They found that rmTBI caused cognitive defects and increased neuronal degeneration, with increased Reactive Oxygen Species (ROS), along with decreased activity of Superoxide Dismutase, Glutathione Peroxidase and Catalase [antioxidants in the body that fight ROS effects]. At the end of the study, they noted: "Our findings confirmed the effect of rosemary extract on improvement of cognitive deficits and suggested its mechanisms might be mediated by anti-oxidative and anti-inflammatory. Therefore, rosemary extract may be a potential treatment to improve cognitive deficits in rmTBI patients."

We have long known that stress both degrades memory and increases reactive oxygen species, so it is hardly surprising that rosemary, which has both stress-reducing effects and antioxidant activity, is able to enhance the memory by reducing stress effects.

Rosemary & Your Eyes

With all its antioxidant and anti-inflammatory effects, we can speculate that rosemary should be helpful in cases of eye troubles, and indeed, it is.

A group of researchers at Wright State University Boonshoft School of Medicine in Dayton, Ohio, investigated some "novel and well-established antioxidants" to see if they would help to slow the progression of the disease in cases of ad-vanced age-related macular degeneration.

The research was done on dark-reared rats that were treated with zinc oxide, or with zinc oxide combined with rosemary powder, or with zinc oxide combined with rosemary oil diluted with polyunsaturated fatty acids. Then the rats were exposed to light. They concluded that the mixture of zinc oxide and rosemary powder was more effective at reducing oxidative stress markers and enhancing visual cell survival.

Therefore, it may help to slow the progression of age-related eye disease.

Scientists at the University of Texas Health Science Center in San Antonio, Texas, looked into some phytochemicals and their effects on photochemical damage. They found that ursolic acid, as contained in rosemary, increased the sensitivity of melanoma cells to ultraviolet radiation and "conferred some photoprotection" to retinal pigment epithelium cells.

Another group of researchers in La Jolla, California, investigated the protective effect of carnosic acid from rosemary on retinal cells treated with hydrogen peroxide to induce oxidative stress, and by giving dark-adapted rats injections of carnosic acid before exposing them to white light.

They discovered that carnosic acid "significantly protected" the retinal cells exposed to oxidative stress. Carnosic acid also protected the rats' retinas from light-induced retinal damage. They concluded that carnosic acid "may potentially have clinical application to diseases affecting the outer retina, including age-related macular degeneration and retinitis pigmentosa, in which oxidative stress is thought to contribute to disease progression."

From these studies, we see that rosemary is indeed beneficial to both the memory and the eyesight.

5: *Rosemary for the Digestion*

Rosemary has long been known as an aid to digestion. Martin de Porres no doubt used the herb with this in mind when he was treating sick patients. Very likely he had a wine-rosemary tonic made up that he dispensed to those he judged needed it. In addition to its other benefits, if rosemary aided a patient's digestion, the patient would improve much faster because of a better intake of nutrients.

Paul Barney, M.D., writes in his book, **Doctor's Guide to Natural Medicine**, that, "Rosemary stimulates bile flow, which improves digestion."

Phyllis A. Balch, CNC, writes in *Prescription for Nutritional Healing, Fifth Edition*, that rosemary "relaxes the stomach."

Both those actions aid a person's digestion.

Researchers at the Al-Fateh University of Medical Sciences in Libya researched the folk medicine uses of rosemary and some of the current research available and concluded that rosemary and its constituents have a potential for use in treatment or prevention of many human disorders, including peptic ulcer.

Interestingly enough, scientists have done a fair amount of research on the effect of rosemary on animal digestion, especially in terms of the effects of the rosemary on the animals' gut flora, which is a major key to animal health.

Since St. Martin de Porres used rosemary to such great benefit in his healing work with animals, this only reaffirms our opinion that rosemary heals "both man and beast."

Gut Health of Sheep

In 2015, Japanese scientists published a study in *Animal Science Journal* in which the researchers evaluated the effects of rosemary essential oil and two types of forage in 48 dairy ewes, looking for differences in the "ewes' performances, immune response and lambs' growth and mortality." They found that rosemary essential oil decreased lamb mortality, improved forage intake and "tended to ameliorate colostrum production; it could be a natural additive to improve ewes' performances."

Since lambs lack an immune system, the rosemary essential oil helped control reactive oxygen species and disease organisms, so that lamb survival and growth was improved overall. The rosemary likely strengthened the animals' ability to stave off disease.

Researchers in 2016 published a study in the *Journal of Animal Science Biotechnology* in which they investigated how adding rosemary leaves to the diet of sheep affects the bacteria living in the animals' rumens, which would consequently have a huge effect on the animals' health.

These scientists checked out the effects of both rosemary leaves added to the animal diets, or rosemary essential oil. They first analyzed the animals' gut contents and quantified the types and amounts of microbial populations. They discovered that the rosemary leaves, either in loose form or in pellet form, "decreased the abundance of archaea and the genus Provatella. The rosemary leaves in loose form also decreased the abundance of Ruminococcus albus and Clostridium aminopilum, while the EO [essential oil] increased the abundance of Fibrobacter succinogenes. The community of bacteria and archaea was not affected by any of the supplements."

Needless to say, this suggests to animal scientists that "rosemary leaves may be used to modulate rumen microbiome and its function," to increase the populations of some desirable species of bacteria and decrease the populations of less desirable bacteria. The microbial population of an animal's rumen is known to aid in the degradation of protein and fiber and likely contributes to the animal's overall nutritional status.

Chicken Digestion & Gut Health

The journal, *British Poultry Science*, published a study that investigated much the same thing as the sheep study above, but in chickens. The researchers checked out the effects of five culinary herbs or their essential oils "on the growth, digestibility and intestinal microflora status in female broiler chicks." The five herbs were thyme, oregano, marjoram, rosemary and yarrow.

The researchers say that thyme and yarrow herb had the most positive effects on chick performance, and no dietary treatment affected the chicks' microflora populations. Rosemary herb affected sialic acid (a monosaccharide that mediates a variety of physiological processes) concentration in a positive way, but rosemary oil caused less sialic acid to be excreted.

They concluded that, "Plant extracts in diets may therefore affect chick performance, gut health and endogenous secretions, although the chemical composition of the extract appears to be important in obtaining the optimal effects."

In the case of chickens, rosemary herb had far more beneficial effects than rosemary oil.

The poultry industry is apparently an up and coming market for rosemary-based dietary treatments, as scientists continue to investigate the effects of various herbs and essential oils on domestic birds. In 2004, scientists studied the "influence of 2 plant extracts on performance, digestibility, and digestive organ weights in broilers." They compared placebo, an essential oil extract from oregano, cinnamon and pepper, and an extract from sage, thyme and rosemary.

They found that "both plant extracts improved the digestibility of the feeds for broilers. The effect of different additives on digestibility improved the performance slightly, but this effect was not statistically significant."

From what we have seen, it is entirely possible that if these scientists had tried dried rosemary leaves, rather than rosemary essential oil, the positive effects might have been greater.

Bioavailability of Nutrients

In 2010, scientists examined whether or not herbs might be a good source of carotenoids (plant pigments with many health benefits for humans), especially if the carotenoids in herbs were more bioaccessible, "using a simulated human in vitro digestion model." They found that, "herbs are rich sources of carotenoids and that these foods can significantly contribute to the intake of bioaccessible carotenoids."

Another study, also done in 2010, involved an antioxidant-enriched extract obtained from rosemary "to be used as an ingredient to design functional foods. The researchers mixed sunflower oil and lecithin with the extract and discovered that, with in vitro digestion, the mixture "reduced by 50% the bioaccesibility in terms of antioxidant activity. Bioavailability was 31%." They apparently concluded that "this activity was not due to the original levels of carnosol, carnosic acid, and methyl carnosate (which only 47% remained after digestion) but due to their derivatives and digestion products."

We concluded that, had these scientists mixed the rosemary extract with something "healthier" than sunflower oil, such as coconut oil, they might have obtained far higher results. Since sunflower oil, a highly unsaturated oil, is a known source of free radicals, the rosemary extract likely wasted a lot of its antioxidant activity on dealing with the known effects of oxygen reacting with the sunflower oil to produce free radicals, a reaction known as lipid peroxidation, or rancidity.

Definitely, rosemary has many properties that aid in human digestion as well as in animal digestion. So far, most of the research seems to show that the whole herb, in dried-leaf form, has the most beneficial effects in animals, and very likely in humans, also.

6: *Rosemary Against Cancer*

The antioxidants and anti-inflammatory constituents of rosemary have a lot to do with the herb's anticancer qualities. Current research shows that rosemary may be a useful addition to an anticancer regime.

We don't think you can go wrong by adding rosemary leaves to your diet now, and maybe you will never have to deal with cancer.

According to the 1999 book, *Professional's Handbook of Complementary & Alternative Medicines*, "In recent years, a number of studies have been published that suggest potential anticancer properties of the plant. These preliminary studies suggest that rosemary components have the potential to decrease activation and increase detoxification of important human carcinogens. Rosemary components might have potential as chemoprotectants, but studies in humans are necessary."

Since that book was written, many more studies have been done that continue to suggest that rosemary may well have a role in cancer prevention and cancer treatment.

For instance, several studies have shown that rosemary or its constituents can inhibit the growth of human cancer cells, such as human myeloid leukemia cells, ER-negative human breast cancer cells, human ovarian cancer cells, colon and pancreatic cancer cells and various others.

In 2001, a group of researchers in Israel investigated carnosic acid derived from rosemary for its strong antioxidant and antimutagenic properties in various cell and animal models. Their study showed that carnosic acid "inhibits proliferation of HL-60 and U937 human myeloid leukemia cells." Anything that slows down cancer cell proliferation slows down the growth of cancer.

According to the researchers, "These results indicate that carnosic acid is capable of antiproliferative action in leuk-emic cells and can cooperate with other natural anticancer compounds in growth-inhibitory and differentiating aspects."

Several American scientists investigated the ability of ex-tracts and purified components of rosemary, including car-nosic acid, to inhibit the growth of human breast cancer cells that were ER-negative, meaning the cancer did not grow in response to estrogen. They treated human breast cancer cells with rosemary/carnosic acid and with tumeric.

They concluded that: "Rosemary/carnosic acid, alone or combined with curcumin, may be useful to prevent and treat ER-negative breast cancer."

Human ovarian cancer cells also experience antiproliferative effects from rosemary extract. Since "recent studies have shown that it has pharmacologic activities for cancer chemo-prevention and therapy," Canadian scientists studied the effects of rosemary extract on human ovarian cancer cells. They showed that the extract "inhibited the proliferation of ovarian cancer cell lines by affecting the cell cycle at multiple phases," and for this reason, rosemary extract "holds pot-ential as an adjunct to cancer chemotherapy."

A group of Spanish researchers in Madrid, aware of the "natural potent antiproliferative" effects of rosemary extracts and its components and in search of a new therapeutic ap-proach to colorectal and pancreatic cancers, investigated rosemary extract for this purpose. They used five different extracts of rosemary in hopes of discovering which strength would be most effective against these cancers. Their results showed that "the antitumor effect of carnosic acid together with carnosol was higher than the sum of their effects separately, which supports the use of the rosemary extract as a whole." They feel that their results "support the use of carnosic-acid-rich rosemary extract as a complementary approach in colon and pancreatic cancer."

As we have previously noted, the whole rosemary herb often appears to work better than extracts that are stronger in one component of the herb. This appears to be what the Spanish scientists discovered.

Three Turkish scientists harvested rosemary leaves from three different locations in Turkey and made extracts from them. They obtained six extracts that were "applied to various human cancer cell lines" that included human small cell lung carcinoma, human liver carcinoma, human chronic myeloid leukemia, and human breast adenocarcinoma. They discovered that the lower concentration extracts resulted in a "superior antiproliferative effect." Thus, "Rosemary extract is a potential candidate to be included in the anti-cancer diet with pre-determined doses avoiding toxicity."

In this particular study, less was definitely more.

Three of the Spanish scientists cited above investigated rosemary further, noting that rosemary "has been reported to possess antitumor activities both in vitro and in animal studies." They reviewed all the available literature in order to summarize "the reported anticancer effects of rosemary," in addition to "the interactions between rosemary and currently used anticancer agents," and go on to discuss "the possibility of using rosemary extract as a complementary agent in cancer therapy" as compared to "its isolated components" such as carnosic acid, carnosol, ursolic acid and rosmarinic acid.

Another group of Spanish researchers decided to find out what compounds in rosemary extract contributed the most to the antiproliferative/cytotoxic effects of rosemary. They discovered that "fractions containing diterpenes or triterpenes were the most active, but not as much as the whole extract." In other words, "the comparative antiproliferative study on the fractions and whole extract revealed potential synergist effects between several components in the extract that may deserve further attention."

Once more, we see that the whole rosemary herb performs better than its parts.

A pair of researchers from the College of Pharmacy, University of Chicago, in 2015 noted that rosemary extracts "standardized to diterpenes (e.g. carnosic acid and carnosol) have been approved by the European Union (EU) and given a GRAS (Generally Recognized as Safe) status in the United States by the Food and Drug Administration." They did a mini-review of the current research on carnosic acid, carnosol, and rosmanol, describing their mechanism of action in different cancers, as these three diterpenes have "received the most attention," with "promising results of anti-cancer activity."

As usual, scientists are determined to find that one factor in the herb that does all the work, probably because they are used to single-chemical drugs. But in the case of rosemary, an herb created by God, the whole herb with all its constituents acting together, will likely continue to outperform each constituent, no matter how powerful.

American scientists in 2014 investigated rosemary extract's effect on androgen receptor degradation, as this is part of the process in prostate cancer. They discovered that the rosemary extract seemed to "preferentially target cancer cells as opposed to 'normal' cells." Furthermore, they believe this herb may be responsible for many of the beneficial effects of the Mediterranean diet. They then add that as rosemary extracts are used as food preservatives in more and more foods, more of the population will be consuming rosemary and receiving benefits far beyond those of the Mediterranean diet by itself.

All this research shows that whole rosemary extracts that contain all the major compounds of rosemary leaves seem to have the most powerful effects against cancer, and do not appear to show any toxic effects.

For general cancer prevention, and even if you are under treatment for some form of cancer, you can't go wrong by including a tablespoon of rosemary leaves in your daily diet.

7: *Rosemary Against Diabetes*

Because it contains such a wide variety of powerfully synergistic anti-inflammatory, antioxidant and anticancer compounds, it is hardly surprising to learn that rosemary also
shows strong blood-sugar-lowering effects, not to mention
kidney-supportive properties and anti-obesity activity, all of
which would be useful to diabetics.

With diabetes now figuring as a national epidemic, as more
and more Americans, even teens, are living on junk-food
diets and are badly overweight, the search is on for natural
compounds that will help in the fight against high blood
sugar and obesity. It appears that rosemary may just be the
item they're looking for.

Mind you, it will be a few years before scientists can publicly
admit this. For one thing, they would put Big Pharma's nose
badly out of joint, and for another, there are not too many
institutions willing to commit money to researchers if a new
moneymaking drug is not likely to be the end product.

So we do not look for a nutraceutical solution to diabetes and
obesity any time soon, even though it may well be right
beneath our collective noses.

With that in mind, let us take a look at some of the ongoing
research into the properties of rosemary and its constituents
against hyperglycemia and how they may work in the body.

Recent Research On Antioxidant Activity

A trio of Italian scientists in 2011 investigated "selected
spices and culinary herbs" to check out "their anti-oxidant
and anti-glycant activities and in vitro inhibitory potential
against enzymes involved in glycemic regulation."

The researchers investigated aqueous and methanol extracts of dry sage, rosemary, basil, parsley, chili, garlic, and onion." They found that the water extracts of rosemary and sage had the most phenolic compounds and "showed the highest ability in binding iron and DPPH (stable free radical molecules), superoxide radicals (another free radical) and advanced glycation end product production (compounds formed when sugar binds with a protein and that contribute to aging and degenerative diseases), lipid peroxidation (rancidity of fats) …"

The aqueous extract was far better at stopping advanced glycation end product formation, and the methanol extracts were better at slowing the production of Amadori compounds (a particular arrangement of a sugar and a protein that is an intermediary in the formation of glycation end products). The authors concluded, "Therefore these spices may be preventive not only against cardiovascular diseases but also type 2 diabetes."

In 2017, Canadian researchers investigated the effects of endurance exercise combined with rosemary leaf extract in diabetic rats. They found that the diabetic rats that got the exercise regimen plus the rosemary extract treatment had "the normal levels of those in the healthy group" in terms of markers for lipid peroxidation." This suggests that endurance exercise plus rosemary extract may enhance antioxidant enzyme activity and decrease lipid peroxidation levels, and thus "may attenuate oxidative stress."

Oxidative stress occurs when the body's defenses against free radicals or reactive oxygen species are less than the amount of free radicals occurring in the body. For a telling look at the results of oxidative stress, view a photograph of the president of the United States at his inauguration and compare it to a photograph taken after a few years in office. Oxidative stress is visible aging.

Tunisian researchers in 2017 investigated the protective effects of rosemary essential oil against oxidative stress in rats. They found that "*Rosmarinus officinalis* essential oils exhibit protective effects" in diabetic rats, "as well as protecting against liver and kidney oxidative stress in rats, reflecting its antioxidant properties."

How Rosemary May Lower Blood Sugar

Several mechanisms have been suggested to explain how rosemary lowers blood sugar.

In 2013, Japanese scientists studied methanol extracts of rosemary and discovered that "the ability of rosemary and its components to suppress cAMP responsiveness of the PEPCK-C or G6Pase gene may contribute to its antihyperglycemic activity." These gene promoters "play a key role in the homeostatic regulation of blood glucose levels," which are "important for managing type II diabetes mellitus."

A study conducted at the University of Illinois in 2014 found that several culinary herbs, including rosemary, appear to "inhibit a molecular target for type 2 diabetes management, dipeptidyl peptidase IV." This is the same target several of the newer diabetes drugs inhibit, so if herbs can do the same thing, then people who cannot afford the expensive drugs can use the herbs. This was the driving idea behind the study.

In 2014, researchers at the University of Dundee in Scotland theorized that carnosic acid, a major constituent of rosemary, "may act to improve glycemic status through enhancing peripheral glucose clearance." In other words, they thought carnosic acid might aid the peripheral muscles of the body—the arms and legs and other skeletal muscle—to burn glucose more efficiently, thus resulting in a lowering of blood sugar.

Their findings "provide new insight into how carnosic acid may improve glucose homeostasis through enhancing peripheral glucose clearance in tissues such as skeletal muscle ... thereby mitigating pathological effects associated with the hyperglycemic state." This means carnosic acid causes the muscles to burn glucose as though they were exercising.

The research also suggests that athletes like long-distance runners or Olympic-style weightlifters may benefit from rosemary to help the muscles burn sugar for energy more efficiently during their long workouts.

Another study, done in 2017 by Canadian investigators, studied rosemary and rosemarinic acid in increasing glucose uptake by skeletal muscles. They found that rosemarinic acid "deserves further study as it shows potential to be used as an agent to regulate glucose homeostasis."

Turkish researchers, noting that rosemary is widely used in Turkish folk medicine for the treatment of high blood sugar, experimented on diabetic rabbits to find the dose of an ethanol (grain alcohol) extract of rosemary that would work best. They found that the highest dose they used was the most effective at lowering the rabbits' blood sugar, and that the higher doses exerted their effects in the company of a significant increase in serum insulin levels in the diabetic rabbits.

In closing, they remark: "It was concluded that probably, due to its potent antioxidant properties, the *Rosmarinus officinalis* extract exerts remarkable antidiabetogenic effect."

Liver & Kidney Protection

It has long been said that your liver is your life. The liver is constantly under assault by much that we eat and definitely by the medications people may take. Anytime someone has a chronic disease such as diabetes, liver protection is doubly important.

In 2013, Saudi Arabian researchers examined the effect of a water extract of rosemary on diabetic rats. They discovered that the rosemary-extract-treated rats had their elevated liver enzymes restored "near to normal" and observed that, "This study revealed that rosemary extracts exerted a hepato-protective effect. The results indicate that the extract exhibits the protective effect on tissues and prove its potentials as an antidiabetic agent."

Scientists working for the McCormick Company's Technical Innovation Center in Maryland published a study in 2013 that "suggested that rosemary potentially increases liver glycolysis and fatty acid oxidation by activating AMPK and PPAR pathways." What this means is that rosemary aided certain important enzymes to function better, so that the liver used glucose and fatty acids better.

Canephron N is an herbal combination that is well known in Europe and Russia and is used for urinary system troubles. It is made of lovage root, rosemary leaves and centaury herb. In 2014, Ukrainian scientists investigated Canephron N for its possible effects on diabetic nephropathy (kidney damage caused by diabetes).

Their results, after six months of therapy combining the Canephron N with standard diabetic treatment and an ACE inhibitor, showed that "the level of microalbuminuria (a moderate increase in the level of albumin protein in the urine that is an early sign of kidney damage) decreased significantly in the study group compared with the control group." Also, "Canephron N had a positive effect on the antioxidant defense status and lipid peroxidation levels." They concluded that Canephron N would be an excellent add-on therapy for patients with diabetic nephropathy.

Naturally, after our studies of rosemary, we feel that much of these good results come from the rosemary in the formula, but if you want to try Canephron N, you can usually find it for sale on eBay out of various European countries.

Rosemary As An Aid In Weight-Loss

Since rosemary is known to help the liver process fats better and burn sugar more efficiently, it is hardly surprising that it would aid in weight loss.

Scientists in Seattle, Washington, investigated carnosic acid isolated from rosemary, as it had been shown to "prevent weight gain and hepatic steatosis (fatty liver)." Since little is known about the safety of carnosic acid at levels high enough to be effective, they decided to investigate hepatotoxicity and cytochrome P450 inhibition and induction. Cytochrome P450 is a family of enzymes chiefly found in the liver, but also in cells all over the body, that are responsible for metabolizing many potentially toxic compounds, including drugs.

Their research showed that there is a potential for carnosic acid to interact with drugs, so they advocate more studies to assess the safety of carnosic acid before it is used as a weight loss aid.

Far better, we feel, to take the rosemary leaves whole, as the carnosic acid probably acts synergistically with the other components of the herb to produce better results all around and with far less danger of interactions.

Iranian scientists in 2016 investigated rosemary as a possible aid in preventing *metabolic syndrome*. Metabolic syndrome is a collection of risk factors occurring in a person that make that person a prime candidate for heart disease and diabetes, not to mention cancer. The risk factors are: elevated blood sugar levels, inflammation, elevated cholesterol and triglycerides, abdominal obesity, bleeding disorders and high blood pressure. This combination of factors is known to raise the risk of diabetes and cardiovascular disease.

The Iranian researchers investigated "the interesting pharmacological effects of rosemary, and its active compounds, and the related mechanisms in the management of the metabolic syndrome that are documented in in vitro and in vivo studies."

To summarize: If you have metabolic syndrome, or if you are at risk for diabetes or fatty liver, or kidney troubles, you can't go wrong by adding rosemary, in the herb form, to your diet. It appears to improve many of the processes that, if unchecked, can lead to these conditions.

Diabetic Ulcers

A Jordanian scientist, knowing that rosemary was used in Jordanian folk medicine for wound management and treatment, conducted a study to check out the healing power of both a water extract of rosemary and the essential oil.

He created wounds on the backs of a number of diabetic rats, which he divided into four groups to compare the two treatments to a group of untreated normal rats and a group of untreated diabetic rats. He observed the wounds for 15 days and measured the rats' blood sugars and body weights and measured the percentage of wound contracture. Not surprisingly, he found that the treated wounds showed reduced inflammation and greater amounts of wound contraction and more regeneration of tissue.

He concluded that: "Results indicated that the essential oil of *Rosmarinus officinalis* was the most active in healing diabetic wounds and provide a scientific evidence for the traditional use of this herb in wound treatment."

It is little wonder that St. Martin de Porres got so much mileage out of one herb, when one considers all the compounds it contains and all the human ailments it works against. His treatment of wounds with wine heated with rosemary has considerable scientific backing.

We feel that this knowledge of how to use rosemary was given by God to St. Martin de Porres.

The regular use of the leaves in the diet also has many benefits.

If people will take rosemary leaf, one tablespoon two times a day, many of their problems will likely be overcome or prevented.

8: *Rosemary For Skin & Hair*

Since rosemary is known to be protective against cancer, it is hardly surprising to learn that it can prevent skin cancers also, when it is used topically and internally. Many experiments have been run in the past few years to explore the ability of rosemary and its constituents to prevent things like ultraviolet light damage to the skin and skin tumors.

Effects on Skin Tumor Formation

In 1994, researchers in New Jersey looked into the effects of an alcohol extract of rosemary on skin tumors. They also experimented with carnosol and ursolic acid isolated from rosemary. What they learned was that application of the rosemary extract to mouse skin five minutes before they applied a carcinogen reduced tumor formation by 54% to 64%, depending upon the strength of the extract. They found that carnosol or ursolic acid also inhibited the number of tumors that would develop on each mouse by 45-61%.

Indian researchers at the University of Rajasthan in 2006 experimented with a rosemary extract, administered orally before mice had tumor-causing and promoting substances applied to their skin. Their results: The average weight and size of tumors were lower in the group of mice treated with rosemary extract. Also, the levels of depleted glutathione in the mice's blood were restored, and the levels of lipid peroxidation (free radical damage) were "significantly reduced" in the mice treated with the rosemary extract.

Italian researchers, recognizing that melanoma skin cancers are on the increase around the world, and that melanoma has a high resistance to cytotoxic agents used in chemotherapy, tested a rosemary hydroalcoholic extract on a human melanoma cell line. They found that the rosemary extract reduced melanoma cell growth in a time and dose-dependent manner. The various dilutions of the extract "drastically reduced cellular metabolic activity." Furthermore, the anti-proliferative (anti-growth) effects of the extract were evident within 24 hours and enhanced at 48 hours and 72 hours of incubation.

The researchers observed that the whole extract of rosemary appeared to have a far greater effect than single components such as carnosol and rosmarinic acid, probably because, as is often the case in herbal medicines, "multi-factorial effects can occur." They concluded: "A 65% (v/v) hydroalcoholic extract of *Rosmarinus officinalis L.* was able to efficiently reduce, in a dose and time dependent manner, the proliferation of the human melanoma A375 cell line, usually highly resistant to cytotoxic agents."

This is great news to us, since very little is known to help against malignant melanoma.

Protection From Ultraviolet Damage

Not surprisingly, researchers have also showed that rosemary has the ability to protect the skin against the aging effects of the sun. Skin has its own complex structure and is vulnerable to free radical damage due to its contact with oxygen and with ultraviolet radiation from sunlight. Since rosemary has strong antioxidant properties, it should help protect against contact with the environment. Studies show that it does.

Spanish and Italian researchers investigated the effects of citrus and rosemary extracts, taken orally, on skin health, in particular for the protection of skin from the harmful effects of UV radiation from the sun. They concluded that the "combination of citrus flavonoids and rosemary polyphenols and diterpenes may be considered as an ingredient for oral photoprotection," and that protection was strongest after 12 weeks of taking the extract.

The same group of researchers investigated the citrus and rosemary combo further about two years later and further stated that "Treated subjects showed a decrease of the UVB- and UVA-induced skin alterations (decreased skin redness and lipoperoxides) and an improvement of skin wrinkledness and elasticity ... Some of the positive effects were noted as short as 2 weeks of product consumption."

Italian scientists, upon observing that reactive oxygen species (free radicals) are thought to be causes of the severe connective tissue damage in several sun-damaged skin problems, decided to treat skin fibroblast cells with a rosemary extract and see if the known antioxidant activity of the rosemary would aid the skin cells in resisting sun damage. They concluded that, "Exogenous supplementation of an anti-oxidant hydrophilic extract from rosemary could have cosmetic benefits and may represent an efficient tool to minimize free radical-induced skin damage." In short, the rosemary extract provided a lot of protection and kept down the damage to the tested skin cells.

In particular, carnosic acid found in rosemary seems to have a lot of potential against sun damage to the skin. Exposing the skin to ultraviolet radiation is known to bring on photoaging in various ways, and some Korean researchers showed that carnosic acid "significantly inhibited" several of the pathways of damage. It also lessened the generation of reactive oxygen species.

A group of Swiss researchers tested various antioxidants for photoprotection abilities and proved that carnosic acid showed "photoprotective potential."

Other Properties Of Rosemary On The Skin

Rosemary not only protects the skin when ingested, but also it protects the skin when used directly on the skin. Various studies point to some interesting properties of the herb when used externally.

A study done by Italian scientists utilized rosemary essential oil loaded into lipid nanoparticles to study some of the effects of the oil applied directly to the skin. They found that this method of applying the essential oil to the skin resulted in significant increases in skin hydration and skin elasticity, which would make it extremely useful for "treatment of cutaneous alterations involving skin hydration and elasticity."

Indeed, oil forms of many nutrients are readily absorbed by the skin. According to Dr. Ray Peat, in his book *Nutrition for Women*, "Oily things enter the body very easily through the skin ... Oily vitamins and hormones can be applied to the skin. Significant quantities of fat (such as olive oil) can be given by massage when the person is too sick to eat." This is known as *skin feeding*.

Some Iranian researchers utilized this property of skin by using rosemary essential oil to aid in carrying a painkiller into the body via the skin and enhancing its effects. They used a diclofenac (an NSAID topical painkiller) gel with three different concentrations of rosemary essential oil and evaluated the pain-killing effects. They concluded that their study "proved the enhancing effect of 0.5 and 1% rosemary essential oil on diclofenac percutaneous (through the skin) absorption."

Turkish researchers investigated whether rosemary extract could help improve skin flap survival when soft-tissue reconstruction work is done. Using rats, they used rosemary oil orally and via subcutaneous injection. They were able to show that "in addition to its anti-inflammatory and anti-oxidant properties, *R. officinalis* has vasodilatory effects that contribute to increased skin flap survival."

Investigators in the Republic of Korea in 2017 looked into carnosol from rosemary and its effect on atopic dermatitis (AD). They found that carnosol has numerous positive effects on the various processes contributing to atopic dermatitis and concluded, "These findings suggest that carnosol exhibited a potential anti-AD activity by inhibiting pro-inflammatory mediators ..." Carnosol treatment reduced skin inflammation considerably.

Rosemary Oil As A Cosmetic Addition

Rosemary essential oil is usually readily available at natural food stores. In addition to the benefits of smelling the oil, it can be added to cosmetics used on your skin, so that you can also get the benefits of its hydrating and antioxidant properties.

Progesterone cream, moisturizer creams, lotions, shampoos ... all can have a few drops of rosemary essential oil added. The oil has so many benefits, any way you can add it to your body is reasonable.

St. Martin's Favorite Remedy

St. Martin de Porres used rosemary in many ways. One of his favorites was to heat rosemary in wine, a fast method of creating an extract, which he then used to cleanse wounds and aid in healing.

Given rosemary's powerful anti-inflammatory effects, its ability to dampen free radical formation, and the fact that it has antibacterial effects, we can see why St. Martin used the herb this way.

We have no doubt that the Holy Spirit guided St. Martin in his use of the items he had available for healing, just as we have no doubt that rosemary possessed all the abilities he needed in a substance he utilized in his chosen profession.

9: *Rosemary As A Food Preservative*

Once we learned that rosemary exerts great activity against food spoilage bacteria, we were hardly surprised that industry is investigating the herb as a possible additive to prepared foods that will aid in extending their shelf life.

Many studies have been made of the herb's antibacterial properties and which bacteria it has the most efficacy against. It is even being considered as an adjunct to regular antibiotic therapy in cases of drug-resistant bacteria infections.

Antibacterial Activity of Rosemary

So many bacteria have grown resistant to antibiotics, researchers are in search of substances that may help in the treatment and prevention of emerging drug-resistant strains of bacteria.

A Polish study in 2013 looked at the essential oils of rosemary and basil against multidrug-resistant strains of *Escherichia coli*. The scientists used clinical strains of the bacteria obtained from patients and equipment with *E. coli* bacteria of various strains. Their results indicate that both oils are active against all the strains of *E. Coli*, including beta-lactamase positive bacteria.

Researchers at the Central Institute of Medicinal and Aromatic Plants in Lucknow, India, discovered that rosemary essential oil was more active against gram-positive pathogenic bacteria, "except *E. faecalis* and drug-resistant mutants of *E. coli*," and also against certain pathogenic fungi and drug-resistant mutants of *Candida albicans*. Their findings suggest that rosemary oil and its constituents "may be useful in counteracting gram-positive bacterial, fungal, and drug-resistant infections."

A follow-up study done by some of the earlier Polish scientists in 2017 sought to determine which essential oils would "support antibiotics against pathogenic bacteria in wounds." They found that rosemary oil was one of the essential oils that had the most additive and synergistic effects against pathogenic bacteria typically found in wounds.

Rosemary Against Food Spoilage

Many researchers have been looking into rosemary's potential as a possible substance for use in extending shelf-life of perishable foods. Since it exhibits activity against various bacteria involved in food spoilage, many studies have been and are being done in this area.

Canadian scientists in 1997 determined that rosemary essential oil was one of four essential oils tested that were most active against two gram-negative and four gram-positive bacteria involved in meat spoilage.

Food scientists in Denmark discovered that dehydrated chicken meat from mechanically deboned chicken necks "can be protected against oxidative deterioration during storage by rosemary extract added to the meat before it was de-hydrated. They found that the rosemary extract did as good a job as the synthetic antioxidants butylated hydroxyanisole and octyl gallate.

These same scientists four years later evaluated rosemary, green tea, coffee and grape skin extracts as preservatives under retail conditions for cooked pork patties. They con-cluded that of these, rosemary "displayed potential for main-taining sensory eating quality in processed pork products."

In other words, it kept the patties fresh and did not cause any changes in taste that would put off customers.

Greek scientists in 2010 studied the effects of adding ground rosemary to rats' diets then administering carbon tetrachloride. They found that the rats that received the ground rosemary before carbon tetrachloride administration had big declines in various markers for liver damage and free radical damage. They concluded that their results, "suggest that dietary rosemary has the potential to become a promising functional food component."

Swiss scientists in 2013 investigated the stability and quality of broiler meat when treated with such things as rosemary leaves, rosehip fruits, chokeberry pomace and nettle. They fed broilers a regular diet with different cages of broilers receiving one of the above additives. When the broilers were analyzed, they checked various markers such as carcass weight, organ weight, skin and liver color and abdominal fat. They discovered that "rosemary is the most suitable dietary antioxidant investigated in this study," although some of the other items "also exhibited interesting properties."

Clearly, rosemary has a promising future as an additive to foods to help prevent spoilage and extend shelf life.

Indeed, a company called Frutarom Food Protection Business Unit in Israel has added an organic rosemary extract to its "oxidation management solutions" line in 2017 that is "designed to prevent oxidation and increase shelf life of food products."

Frutarom says it "sought expertise in growing organic rosemary and incorporating its active ingredients, carnosic and rosmarinic acids, into food formulation to naturally increase shelf life of foods and beverages." By collaborating with farmers in Spain and Hishtil Nurseries in Israel, they believe they have created "a sustainable supply chain for this 'farm-to-fork' organic product."

It is only a matter of time until we begin seeing products on grocery store and natural foods store shelves that incorporate this particular ingredient as a food preservative.

10: *Possible Adverse Reactions*

The rosemary herb has so many great properties, we can't help but think it perfect—a substance with no adverse effects.

The fact is, however, that any substance, no matter how beneficial it is to almost all people, will not be handled well by certain other individuals.

Avoid High Dosages

Moreover, as we observed earlier, rosemary seems to work best in its herb form, as all its constituents are present, and not in overpowering doses. In many experiments we looked at, rosemary worked best (1) as the whole herb and (2) in lower doses rather than higher.

Indeed, high doses of rosemary can cause vomiting, spasms, pulmonary edema, miscarriage and coma.

Miscarriage and Other Pregnancy Problems

Rosemary has long been known to cause problems in pregnancy. It is said that a pregnant woman should not use rosemary, except as a normal seasoning in cooking. Effects are unknown in breastfeeding women, so again, avoid use of the herb or essential oil for medicinal purposes both during pregnancy and during breastfeeding.

Rosemary oil may have antifertility effects, according to Daniel Mowrey in *Proven Herbal Blends*, and "may prevent implantation but does not appear to interfere with the normal development of the fertilized ova after implantation (Lemonica et al., 1996)."

Mowrey also advises that the undiluted oil of rosemary should not be taken internally until its safety can be verified.

Drug Interactions

Rosemary in higher doses can interfere with the actions of certain drugs. Among them are:

Anticoagulant drugs, such as Warfarin and Clopidogrel.

Blood pressure drugs of the ACE-inhibitor class, such as Zestril (lisinopril), Monopril (fosinopril), Capoten) captpril and Vasotec (elaropril).

Diuretics, such as hydrocholothiazide (HCTC) and Lasix (furosemide).

Lithium, used to treat bipolar disorder. Rosemary apparently may act as a diuretic and cause lithium to reach toxic levels.

A special warning is in order for persons taking *Disulfiram*, a drug used to treat chronic alcoholism. Rosemary in its herbal form or as tablets would probably not interact, but if these people take even small amounts of a rosemary tincture, where the rosemary constituents have been extracted by alcohol, they can experience all the ill effects Disulfiram is supposed to cause when alcohol is consumed.

Adverse Reactions

Rosemary itself can cause problems in certain people who are sensitive to it. In addition to the anti-fertility effects it may cause, it can cause the usual allergic responses in susceptible people.

It may cause dermatitis (skin reactions) and photosensitivity (sunburn after a short time spent in the sun that usually causes the person no problems).

It may cause erythema, or reddening of the skin, and rash-ing, usually with products meant for skin or bath use.

Rosemary oil should not be used in persons with epilepsy. It may trigger seizures in some people.

Large doses of the essential oil may cause stomach and intestinal irritation and kidney damage.

Recent Studies

A 2006 study published in the journal *Contact Dermatitis* notes that there are several reported cases of contact dermatitis with rosemary. The Spanish researchers reported on the case of a man with several episodes of an itchy red rash that resulted in peeling of his skin after using rosemary alcohol on his chest. They found that he also reacted to other plants in the labiate family that rosemary belongs to.

Canadian researchers reported in the journal, *Allergy*, on a person with occupational asthma "caused by several aromatic herbs: thyme, rosemary, bay leaf, and garlic." They concluded that these herbs, including rosemary, "should be included among agents causing occupational asthma in the food industry."

So there we have it. Just as with any other substance, no matter how beneficial, there are always certain people who should not take it, and in rare cases, should not even touch it.

11: *Hair Growth & Cosmetic Use*

Recipes for shampoos and hair rinses incorporating rosemary have been popular for centuries, because rosemary is known to be helpful both for growing hair and for giving dark hair shine and vigor. Old herbal remedy books say that it improves scalp circulation and even fights early graying of hair.

Rosemary essential oil, applied directly to the scalp, stimulates hair growth and helps prevent hair from falling out. It also helps to treat dandruff, because of its antibacterial and antifungal qualities.

Rosemary oil may be good for alopecia (hair loss) in men that is thought to be a result of testosterone being turned into DHT, also known as male pattern baldness. A 2015 study done by researchers in Iran compared rosemary oil treatment to minoxidil treatment to two groups of fifty men. They found that rosemary oil did just as well as minoxidil in treating male pattern baldness, but without the side effect of itchy scalp that plagued the minoxidil group.

This treatment takes some time, however. At three months into the study, the scientists checked and found no growth with either treatment. At six months, both the rosemary group of men and the minoxidil group had "significant increases" in hair growth.

If you wish to try rosemary for hair growth, you can massage rosemary essential oil directly onto the scalp, or if you have sensitive skin, you can dilute the rosemary essential oil in a carrier oil, such as olive oil. Simply add 3 to 5 drops of rosemary oil to a tablespoon of olive oil.

Alopecia can be caused by problems other than male pattern baldness, such as autoimmune diseases. In these cases, rosemary might not help, but it is certainly worth a good trial. A 1998 study done by Scottish researchers involved a randomized, double-blind trial with 86 patients who had been diagnosed with alopecia areata, an autoimmune disorder that causes hair loss.

The patients were divided into two groups, one of which used only carrier oils such as jojoba or grapeseed, as a daily scalp massage. The other group used the carrier oil combined with essential oils of thyme, rosemary, lavender and cedarwood. At the end of 7 months, 44% of the patients in the essential oil group showed improvement, as compared to 15% of the patients in the control group who used only the carrier oils. The researchers concluded that treatment with the essential oils was "significantly more effective" than treatment with the carrier oil alone.

It looks to us as though that daily scalp massage probably had a lot to do with that 15% improvement in the control group. When you combine rosemary oil with the daily scalp massage, your chances of good results increase greatly.

If you have alopecia of any variety, we recommend that you combine a daily scalp massage with rosemary oil with a good rosemary shampoo and a rosemary rinse. Don't look for overnight results. Give the treatment at least six months to show its effects.

Rosemary For Hair Maintenance

Rosemary can be added to your current shampoo in the form of rosemary essential oil. You will only need a few drops for this purpose, as a drop of the essential oil goes quite a long way. This probably works best if your shampoo has a scent that goes well with rosemary, such as mint.

If you'd rather make your own shampoo, one method is to buy a bottle of liquid castile soap, available at natural foods stores or certain grocery stores. Pick an unscented soap if possible, or any other scent you'd like that will blend well with rosemary. Add rosemary essential oil until you like the scent and mix well.

Another method is to pour the castile soap into a saucepan and a cup or two of very strong rosemary tea. To make a strong rosemary tea, bring two cups of water to a boil and pour it over two tablespoons of rosemary herb. Let the mixture steep for a good twenty minutes, then strain out the rosemary and add the tea, also known as an *infusion*, to the castile soap in the saucepan. Stir the mixture over low heat until the tea and the castile soap are well blended. Remove from heat and add, if desired, a few drops of rosemary essential oil. Stir to incorporate.

When the mixture is thoroughly cooled, pour it into bottles, and seal them tightly. Store the bottles in a cool, dark place until you are ready to use them.

A good hair rinse is made by pouring one cup of boiling water over 3 tablespoons of rosemary and simmering gently for about 5 minutes. Strain out the rosemary and blend this infusion with a cup of distilled or very pure water. After you have shampooed and rinsed your hair well, pour this mixture through your hair as a finishing rinse. Do not rinse it out. Simply towel your hair and dry it as usual.

Many people like the squeaky-clean feel of a vinegar rinse for their hair. Make yours by adding 1/2 cup of distilled water and ½ cup of vinegar to the infusion above. You will receive the benefits of both the vinegar and the rosemary.

Rosemary Bath Soap

If you enjoy making your own natural soaps, Dr. "B"s soap recipe for a delicious-smelling rosemary soap is as follows:

Dr. "B"s Extra Fine Rosemary Soap

Ingredients:

42 ounces coconut oil

16 ounces lard or Palm oil

6 ounces olive oil

9 ounces caustic soda; dry lye flakes or powder

27–28 ounces distilled water

3 ounces pure cocoa butter

6 ounces Rosemary essential oil

4 tablespoons finely chopped rosemary herb

1 to 2 tablespoons Borax

4 – 250 mg capsules BHT (if available)

Equipment:

Large sturdy plastic stir spoon; 32–oz. heat–proof glass (Pyrex measuring cup) container for lye solution; measuring spoons; rubber gloves; eye goggles; molds; large glass or stainless steel U–bowl (4–6 quart size); two good laboratory measure thermometers; scale for ounces and pounds.

Directions:

Put goggles and gloves on. Have vinegar or lemon juice close by to douse with if any lye solution gets on skin. Melt lard if using this. Pour all oils into large U–bowl, except essential oil and cocoa butter. Stir and set aside and bring to 100 degrees F. Melt cocoa butter. Combine essential oil and cocoa butter in small measuring cup; set aside.

Place Pyrex measuring cup in ice water bath; add water; measure out lye flakes. Pour lye flakes/powder slowly into cold water, stirring constantly but not briskly. When all lye has been poured and incorporated into the cold water, add borax and continue stirring periodically with large, heavy duty plastic spoon. Place thermometer in lye solution and bring to 100 degrees F. When both solutions, *lye and oil*, are close to the required temperature, remove the lye from ice water bath; gently and carefully dry bottom of Pyrex container.

Now comes the fun part: You are ready to make **Soap**--this is the *saponification* process when the lye solution is mixed with the oils and starts making. Slowly, add the lye solution to the oil mixture as you stir in a gentle figure eight pattern. Stir for 20 minutes; then periodically, for several more hours, as the solution begins to thicken and leave a trace on top when the spoon is removed and drizzled across the surface of the amalgam. An electric egg beater set on *very low* can decrease time considerably. Take care not to splash or splatter.

When the trace is thick and takes a few seconds to sink back into the solution, add the essential oil combination and continue stirring periodically as the saponification is going more to completion. If you have them, open the butylated hydroxyltoluene antioxidant capsules (BHT) and pour contents into the amalgam. Throw away the empty capsules. The BHT stops the soap from going rancid. The free fatty acids will work for you and not against you. When a thick trace is evident, pour the mixture into molds.

Be cautioned not to leave your amalgam unattended while it is saponifying. It resembles pastry cream, cake batter, etc., and small children could try sampling it from the bowl with disastrous results. Don't even have them present while making soap, unless behind you at a safe distance from any inadvertent splatters. Clean up preparation materials immediately as they may try to lick the bowls, spoons, and so forth. Be extremely cautious around small children. It is best not to even have them near!

Mold Preparation:

Anything will do, that you want your soap to be shaped as; or you can use a square wooden or plastic box, 14 x 10 inches. Just don't use aluminum, iron, tin, or Teflon, as lye corrodes them. Use wood, glass, enamel or stainless steel. Line your mold with two layers of wax paper. Allow it to flow over the sides of the mold. This facilitates easy removal.

After the soap has been poured into the mold, place the mold in a relatively warm, dry place and cover with cardboard or a wooden cover cut to fit your square box. Individual molds can be covered collectively with one large cardboard. Then, cover with a heavy blanket or several old towels. This allows the heat of reaction to rise and react more fats with the lye. It is still very caustic at this point.

After 72 hours, the soap is ready for removal and cutting into bars. Cut your soap bars into the size you desire and place them in another large wooden or cardboard box. Cover the box with a linen cloth to allow the soap to get even more mild—more base (any unreacted lye) is given a chance to react with any fatty acid esters left or free fatty acids. Let your soap cure for three to six weeks this way. Turn the bars over once during the curing time.

Once your soap has cured for several weeks, then wrap each bar in tissue type paper. Store in a dry, cool cupboard for future use.

The recipe we have given is a *superfatted* soap that makes a mild bath and cleansing bar, also with antiseptic, preservative, and cleansing qualities. Superfatted soaps incorporate oils that are excess to the recipe. They are added last (essential oils and cocoa butter) so they do not all react and become saponified; thus enriching the emollient qualities of the soap. They also *mild* the soap from any free lye that may not have reacted. This is why you want BHT antioxidant to keep the free fat from becoming rancid. We like superfatted soaps for these and other reasons.

The rosemary essential oil and rosemary herb give this particular soap even more antiseptic and antifungal qualities, not to mention the stimulating scent of rosemary it exudes.

12: *Rosemary Recipes*

Rosemary is an extremely versatile herb, useful in cooking, in cosmetics, and in herbal medicine. Following are some suggestions for using rosemary as a health treatment and in cooking.

Rosemary Tinctures

Many people like to make their own herbal *tinctures*. A tincture is defined to be a medicine created when a drug is dissolved in alcohol. An old-fashioned and inexpensive way to make a tincture is to steep a medicinal herb in a bottle of wine.

You can easily make your own rosemary tinctures in this way, as rosemary goes well in either red or white wine.

Buy a bottle of inexpensive wine of your choice. Open the top and pour out a couple of ounces of the wine. Using a funnel, add 3 or 4 tablespoons of rosemary herb, finely chopped. Re-cap the bottle and let it sit for several days to a week. Strain out the rosemary herb. Wash out the wine bottle and, using your funnel, return the strained wine tincture to its bottle. Keep the bottle in a cool, dry place, such as a kitchen cupboard, and take about one tablespoon per day.

Another excellent treatment for body aches is a tincture made by using a tablespoon of finely chopped rosemary in a 375 mL (about 1 pint) bottle of Everclear (pure grain alcohol, also known as *ethanol*). Pour out a little of the Everclear and add the rosemary. Cap the bottle and let it sit in a cool, dry place for about a week. Then strain out the rosemary and either return the tincture to the rinsed Everclear bottle or place it in a spray bottle.

Some people use the spray bottle to apply the rosemary to different areas of their body. Others splash it on directly from the Everclear bottle. Any method you choose is fine.

Recipes Featuring Rosemary

LaRousse Gastronomique, a encyclopedia of cooking techniques and ingredients that is well-known in culinary circles, gives the following summary of rosemary as an ingredient in cooking:

"An aromatic shrub native to Mediterranean countries, whose evergreen leaves are used either fresh or dried as a flavoring. As they have a very pungent taste, only a few leaves are needed to flavor a marinade, a ragout, a game dish, or a grill. The name comes from the Latin *rosmarinus* (rose of the sea) and the herb combines particularly well with veal; it is also used in some tomato sauces and with oven-cooked fish. In northern Europe it is used to flavor sausage meat, sucking pig, and roast lamb. In addition, a sprig of rosemary gives a delicate flavor to the milk used for a dessert. The flowers can be used to garnish salads and they can be crystallized (candied) in the same way as violet. Rosemary honey, a specialty of Narbonne in France, is much esteemed."

For this reason, many, many recipes feature rosemary as one of the spices in meat, lamb, poultry and fish dishes. No doubt you already have a favorite of your own. The following are some of Dr. "B"s favorites.

Skewers of Lamb With Herbs

½ leg of lamb, boned

½ medium onion

1 clove garlic

6 sprigs lemon thyme

6 sprigs marjoram

3 sprigs lovage

3 sprigs rosemary

3 sprigs parsley

½ cup olive oil

½ cup red wine

Cut the meat into cubes about 1 inch square and pour them in a bowl. Peal the onion, slice it thinly and mix with the meat. Stir in the peeled and crushed garlic. Pick the leaves of the herbs off their branches and chop. Mix with the meat. Stir in the oil and the wine. Leave for 4 to 6 hours or overnight.

Thread the pieces of meat loosely on to skewers. Cook over charcoal or an open fire, or grill (broil). Use the remaining marinade for basting. If you have plenty of rosemary, burn some sprigs under the skewers and use a little branch as a basting brush. Serve immediately, with fried rice and a mixed salad.

Veal With Rosemary

½ onion

3 tablespoons olive oil

2 cloves garlic

2 lbs lean veal, from the leg

Sea salt and black pepper

½ lb fresh tomatoes or 14 oz. can tomatoes, drained

½ cup dry white wine

3 sprigs rosemary

Peel and chop the onion. Heat the oil in a saucepan and cook the onion gently until pale golden. Peel and crush the garlic and add it to the onion while it is cooking. Cut the meat into neat rectangular pieces and add them to the pan. Stir around until browned on all sides. Add salt and black pepper. Peel and deseed the tomatoes; chop them quite finely and add to the pan. (If using canned tomatoes, drain off the juice, chop the tomatoes roughly, and add to the meat.) Pour on the wine, put in the sprigs of rosemary and cover the pan. Cook gently for 1 ½ hours, stirring occasionally. To serve the veal stew, take out the rosemary and accompany with rice and a green salad.

Hot or Deviled Lamb

2 lb. boneless lean lamb, cubed

salt and pepper

¼ tsp cayenne pepper

½ cup olive oil

2 garlic cloves, chopped

2 tsp chopped fresh rosemary

1 cup white wine

Season the meat with salt, pepper and cayenne, and brown it in a frying pan with the oil, garlic and rosemary. Cook over high heat, shaking the pan frequently to avoid sticking.

When the lamb is golden brown, add the wine and cook uncovered until the wine evaporates. Serve immediately.

Veal in Milk

2 lb. boned veal shoulder, in 1 piece

5 tbsp. butter

fresh rosemary

fresh sage

18 small boiling onions

salt and freshly ground white pepper

grated nutmeg

1 ½ quarts milk

Spread 4 tablespoons of the butter inside the bottom of a roasting pan, rub the veal with the rest of the butter and place the veal in a pan along with a few sprigs of rosemary and some sage leaves. Put the pan in an oven, preheated to 400 degrees F, for 30 minutes. Turn frequently and baste the veal from time to time with the meat juices.

Remove the bouquet garni (herbs) and put the veal in an ovenproof dish with a tightly fitting lid. Garnish the meat with onions and season it with salt, pepper and a pinch of nutmeg. Boil the milk and add enough to cover the ingredients. Put the lid on the dish and cook the veal in the oven at 350 degrees F for 2 hours. Remove the meat, slice and arrange it in a warmed, shallow serving dish. Sieve the cooking liquid and pour it over the slices of veal. Serve hot.

Roast Chicken With Rosemary

1 three-pound chicken, whole

salt and pepper

1 onion, cut into quarters

¼ cup fresh rosemary, chopped

Rinse chicken well and season with salt and pepper. Stuff the cavity with the onion and rosemary and place chicken in a 9 x 13-inch baking dish Place into an oven that has been pre-heated to 350 degrees F and cook for 2 ½ hours, or until chicken is thoroughly cooked and juices run clear.

Rosemary Quick Bread

1 tablespoon sugar

1 cup warm (not hot) water

1 package (0.25 oz) active dry yeast

1 teaspoon salt

2 tablespoons butter, softened

2 tablespoons finely chopped rosemary

1 teaspoon Italian seasoning

3 cups bread flour

1 tablespoon olive oil

1 egg, beaten

Dissolve the sugar in warm water in a bowl and mix in the yeast. When yeast is bubbly, add salt, butter, 1 tablespoon rosemary and Italian seasoning. Mix in 2 cups of flour. Gradually add the remaining flour to form a dough and knead 10 to 12 minutes.

Coast the inside of a large bowl with olive oil. Place dough in bowl and cover. Allow to rise for 1 hour in a warm location.

Punch down dough and divide in half. Line a baking sheet with parchment paper and lightly grease paper. Shape dough into two round loaves and place on the baking sheet. Sprinkle with the remaining rosemary. Cover and allow to rise for 1 hour, until loaves have doubled in size.

Brush loaves with egg if desired. Bake 15 to 20 minutes, or until golden brown.

Mashed Potatoes & Yams With Rosemary

6 to 8 cloves garlic, unpeeled

3 tablespoons olive oil

1 ½ cups backing potatoes, peeled and cubed

1 ½ cups yams, peeled and cubed

½ cup milk

¼ cup butter

½ tsp. dried rosemary

½ cup grated Parmesan cheese

salt and pepper

Place garlic in a small ovenproof bowl and drizzle with olive oil. Roast for 30 minutes in an oven preheated to 350 degree F for 30 minutes, or until very soft. Cool and peel garlic and reserve the oil.

Boil potatoes and yams in a large pot of salted water until tender, about 20 minutes. Drain and reserve 1 cup of liquid.

Place potatoes and yams in a large bowl with milk, butter, rosemary, garlic and reserved olive oil. Mash to desired consistency, adding reserved cooking liquid as required. Mix in ¼ cup of Parmesan cheese. Season with salt and pepper. Transfer to an 8-inch square, lightly greased baking dish. Sprinkle with remaining cheese.

Bake until thoroughly heated and golden on top, about 45 minutes.

Rosemary-Flavored Butter & Oil

Many cooks make a long-lasting, rosemary-infused olive oil by placing a tablespoon of dried rosemary leaves into olive oil and letting it sit for two weeks in the sun. After two weeks, strain out the rosemary and store the oil in the pantry. It will last a year.

A delicious rosemary butter consists of ½ cup of butter, softened, mixed with 3 teaspoons finely chopped fresh rosemary or 1 teaspoon dried rosemary. Thoroughly mix the two ingredients then spoon the mixture onto a sheet of parchment paper. Roll the paper into a log shape and twist the ends to seal. Refrigerate the log for at least 3 hours until firm. To serve, cut thin rounds from the log.

Rosemary Honey

Make your own rosemary honey the fast way or the slow way. If you prefer natural, raw honey, make yours the slow way so you won't destroy any of the natural enzymes raw honey contains.

For a naturally infused rosemary honey, use 3 parts raw honey to 1 part of rosemary. Combine them in a jar and use a knife to push the rosemary down into the honey and remove as much trapped air as possible. Allow the jar to sit for 2 to 6 weeks then strain out the rosemary using a mesh strainer.

For a quick rosemary honey, heat to a simmer 1 cup of honey with 5 rosemary sprigs in a small saucepan. Simmer for 5 minutes then allow the mixture to cool. Remove the rosemary and transfer the honey to a jar.

13: *How To Grow Your Own Rosemary*

Many people grow rosemary in small potted herb gardens on their window sills in order to have fresh rosemary available when they want it. But rosemary is such a hardy plant, especially in the southern regions of the United States, that it can be easily grown outdoors.

Rosemary is susceptible to cold weather, as it originated in the Mediterranean area, but it can withstand short freezes. According to Burpee Seeds and Plants Company, if your area has sustained temperatures during the winter below 30 degrees F, grow your rosemary in pots that can be moved indoors.

You can successfully grow rosemary in pots inside or outside on patios or terraces, in window boxes, in container gardens and even in hanging baskets.

A typical rosemary bush can grow up to four feet high and spread out four feet on all sides. If you decide to have a plant in your garden, be sure to allow it enough space. Rosemary is often used in landscaping, so if you plant a row, be sure to allow two to three feet between the plants.

Rosemary is one of those plants that can be "trained" into certain shapes. One Christmas staple at nurseries are rosemary plants that have been shaped into miniature Christmas trees, also known as *cone trees*. You can pick up well-started plants during the Christmas season if you find a nursery selling cone trees.

Planting Rosemary

Rosemary does not start well from seed. Your best bet is to pick up a plant from the local nursery, or order plants from a mail-order nursery or even Amazon.com, and set it out in your garden. Choose a spot that gets full sun and that is well-drained does not get a sustained wind or catch a lot of water during a rain.

Rosemary grows slowly for the first year, but by years two and three, it seems to take hold and begins to grow. By year three or four, you may have a full-sized rosemary bush in your garden.

When you want fresh rosemary, clip the new growth, as these sprigs yield the best flavor.

You can keep your rosemary plant trimmed so long as you don't cut back more than a third of the plant at any one time. When you trim, cut branches just above a leaf joint. Usually, the best time to trim back your plant is after it has flowered.

Rosemary planted in pots can become root bound once it begins to grow well, and you may see yellowing of the lower foliage. When this happens, the plant need to be transferred into a larger pot.

Once your rosemary is in the ground or the pot, it usually needs little attention. This is an herb that adapts well to dry conditions. It will thrive so long as it gets the sunlight it craves. In fact, rosemary that is over-watered may wind up with brown leaves.

What Variety Is Best?

Rosemary comes in many varieties, with various colors of flowers. There are even creeping varieties that hug the ground for those who want more ground cover.

If you intend to harvest your plant to use in cooking, cooks tend to prefer these varieties:

Benendon Blue

Flora Rosa

Hill Hardy

Huntington Carpet

Irene

McConnell's Blue

Majorca Pink

Miss Jessup

Tuscan Blue

Spice Island

These tend to be large, upright plants, which are easier to harvest, four to six feet in the ground, with large, fragrant leaves that hold flavor well when cooked or dried.

When To Prune Rosemary

Rosemary can be pruned as often as once a month if you are trying to control the size of the plant. Most people prefer to prune their plants once a year after the plant has flowered. Once the plant has been pruned, you can apply fertilizer or compost. Rosemary does not require constant fertilizing and is usually only fertilized once a year.

When pruning, do not remove more than one-third of the plant and cut branches just above a leaf joint, as described earlier.

Starting New Plants

Rosemary is hard to start from seed, so if you want to give plants to your friends, your best bet is to use cuttings from your own rosemary bush. Once your plant is growing well, you can start new rosemary plants from stem cuttings or from root cuttings.

To start a new plant from stem cuttings, simply snip a two- to six-inch cutting from a new-growth stem and strip the leaves from the bottom half of the stem. Dip the bottom half in rooting hormone (available from plant nurseries and garden stores) and plant it in a container of starting mix. Place the container in a warm area in direct sun. Mist it daily and keep the soil damp. In two to three weeks, check your cuttings for new root growth.

Once your cuttings have roots, they can be transferred to pots, or even transplanted outside if you have a good growing area for rosemary.

If you have a large, hardy plant, new rosemary plants may be started from root cuttings in the fall of the year. Expose a few roots, and select a larger root from ¼ to ½ inches in diameter. Cut it off near the plant and dig it out, then fill in the hole with soil. Cut the root into two-inch sections and trim off the branch roots.

Lay the sections on top of moist rooting medium and cover lightly with rooting medium. Put the tray you are using into a clear plastic bag and set it in indirect light or fluorescent light. Remove the bag for about one hour each day.

The root sections should begin to root and shoot up a stem in about two or three months. Transfer to pots, then in spring you can transfer the new plants to pots or to your garden.

Harvesting Rosemary

Most cooks prefer to use fresh rosemary, as the taste is considered superior to any other form.

When you cut stems off your plant for use in your kitchen, you will quickly see why the upright plants are easier to harvest than a variety that hugs the ground. The younger stems and leaves yield the best taste, so harvest only the new growth.

Rosemary can be harvested at any time of the day and lose none of its taste, although many suggest harvesting in the morning hours is best.

Preparing Rosemary For Use

If you intend to use your rosemary fresh, store it in a plastic bag and do not wash the stems until you are ready to use them.

If you wish to keep a supply of fresh rosemary always on hand, you can freeze the herb. In this case, wash the harvested stems, drain them, and air dry. Leave the leaves on the stem until you are ready to use them.

Freezing rosemary yields a product with taste that is the most like the fresh herb. Frozen rosemary keeps well for years and loses very little taste. The only problem is that freezing softens the herb.

Most people are familiar with the dried rosemary leaves purchased in spice bottles in the grocery store. Drying is the time-honored way of preserving the herb for later use, and it results in surprisingly little loss of taste.

Air Drying

When you harvest rosemary stems, bundle them together and tie them near the bottoms of the stems. Rinse them and shake dry. Hang the stems in an area of low humidity, where the temperature remains around 90 to 120 degrees F.

Once more, leave the leaves on the stems until you are ready to use them. Dried herbs are usually good for one year. After that, they deteriorate and lose flavor.

Oven Drying

If you live in a high-humidity area or otherwise have a reason for wanting your rosemary dried quickly, you can utilize either your oven or your microwave oven to quick-dry your herbs.

To oven-dry, wash and dry your rosemary stems first, then spread them on a cookie sheet. If using a gas oven, the heat of the gas pilot is often enough to dry the herbs well. Check in 2 to 3 hours, and if the herbs appear to be drying, keep them in the oven for up to 12 hours.

In an electric oven, you may need to leave the oven door open and put the oven on its lowest setting. Proper drying should take several hours.

To dry your rosemary in a microwave oven, put 4 or 5 stems on a double thickness of paper towels. Cover with a single towel and microwave at full power for 2 to 3 minutes, until the leaves are brittle. If the leaves are not yet brittle, microwave again for another 30 seconds.

Remember, in growing and preserving your own rosemary herb, you are saving a lot of money that you would have spent at the grocery store, especially if you use a lot of rosemary in your cooking.

Figuring up the amount of money you've saved over buying lots of those small spice bottles of rosemary from the grocery store can cheer up an otherwise dreary day.

Adding Rosemary To Your Diet

If you desire to add rosemary to your diet in order to gain some of its benefits for your health, there are several ways you can do so.

Rosemary Herb

You can always buy rosemary in bottles at the grocery store or in bulk packages of about one pound at natural foods stores. Take about 1 tablespoon per day, either mixed into a soft food or chewed and swallowed. Rosemary can be a bit rough to chew, but if you keep it moistened while chewing, it is relatively pleasant tasting and easy to eat.

Rosemary Capsules

Capsules of rosemary, both in natural form and in dried-extract form are available in natural foods stores. Take up to six per day of the regular capsules and around 3 a day of the extract, which tends to be stronger.

Rosemary Tea

Natural foods stores also carry rosemary tea, usually in bags. You can brew up two to three cups per day if desired.

Rosemary Tincture

Many people like to make their own rosemary tinctures by adding a couple of tablespoons of rosemary to a bottle of wine and letting it sit for a week or so. Take about 1 tablespoon per day of this as a tonic for the body.

Resources

All About Herbs, James McNair, Ortho Books, 1990.

Allergy*, Occupational Asthma Caused by Aromatic Herbs,* Lemiere C, Cartier A, Lehrer SB, Malo JL, September 1996.

***Alternative Therapies in Health and Medicine** , Potential of Rosemary Oil to be Used in Drug-Resistant Infections,* Luqman S, Dwivedi GR, Darokar MP, Kalra A, Khanuja SP, September-October, 2007.

Animal Science Journal, *Effects of Rosmarinus officinalis L. Essential Oils Supplementation on Digestion, Colostrum Production of Dairy Ewes and Lamb Mortality and Growth,* Smeti S, Joy M, Hajji H, Munoz F, Mahouachi M, Atti N, July 2015.

Archives of Dermatology*, Randomized Trial of Aromatherapy. Successful Treatment for Alopecia Areata,* Hay IC, Jamieson M, Ormerod AD, November, 1998.

Balkan Medical Journal*, Use of Systemic Rosmarinus officinalis to Enhance the Survival of Random-Pattern Skin Flaps,* Ince B, Bilgen F, Gundeslioglu AO, Dadaci M, Kozacioglu S, November 2016.

Beef & Veal, The Good Cook: Techniques & Recipes Series, Editors of Time-Life Books, 1979.

Biomolecules & Therapeutics*, Inhibitory Effect of Carnosol on Phthalic Anhydride-Induced Atopic Dermatitis Via Inhibition of STAT3,* Lee DY, Hwang CJ, Choi JY, Park MH, Oh KW, Son DJ, Lee SH, Han SB, Hong JT, September 2017.

Burns, *The Ability of Selected Plant Essential Oils to Enhance the Action of Recommended Antibiotics Against Pathogenic Wound Bacteria*, Sienkiewicz M, Lysakowska M, Kowalczyk E, Szymanska G, Kochan E, Krukowska J, Olszewski J, Zielinska-Blizniewska H, March 2017.

Canadian Journal of Diabetes, *Beneficial Effects of Endurance Exercise with Rosmarinus officinalis Labiatae Leaves Extract on Blood Antioxidant Enzyme Activities and Lipid Peroxidation in Streptozotocin-Induced Diabetic Rats*, Nazem F, Farhangi N, Neshat-Gharamaleki M, June, 2015.

Cancer Letters, *Diterpenes from Rosemary (Rosmarinus officinalis): Defining Their Potential for Anti-Cancer Activity*, Petiwala SM, Johnson JJ, October 2015.

Cancer Research, *Inhibition of Skin Tumorigenesis by Rosemary and Its Constituents Carnosol and Ursolic Acid*, Huang MT, Ho CT, Ferraro T, Lou YR, Stauber K, Ma W, Georgiadis C, Laskin JD, Conney AH., February 1994.

Cell Signal, *Carnosic Acid Stimulates Glucose Uptake in Skeletal Muscle Cells Via a PME-1/PP2A/PKB Signaling Axis*, Lipina C, Hundal HS, November 2014.

Contact Dermatitis, *Rosemary Contact Dermatitis and Cross-Reactivity With Other Labiate Plants*, Gonzalez-Maheve I, Lobesa T, Del Pozo MD, Blasco A, Venturini M, April 2006.

Current Neurovascular Research, *The Cellular Protective Effects of Rosmarinic Acid: From Bench to Bedside*, Nabavi SF, Tenore GC, Daglia M, Loizzo MR, Nabavi SM, 2015.

Drug Metabolism Disposition, *In Vitro Hepatotoxicity and Cytochrome P450 Induction and Inhibition Characteristics of Carnosic Acid, a Dietary Supplement with Antiadipogenic Properties*, Dickmann LJ, VandenBrink BM, Lin YS, July 2012.

Experimental Dermatology, *Carnosic Acid, A Phenolic Diterpene from Rosemary, Prevents UV-Induced Expression of Matrix Metalloproteinases in Human Skin Fibroblasts and Keratinocytes*, Park M, Han J, Lee CS, Soo BH, Ha H, May 2013.

Experimental Gerontology, *Protective Effect of Supercritical Fluid Rosemary Extract, Rosmarinus officinalis, on Antioxidants of Major Organs of Aged Rats*, Posadas SJ, Caz V, Largo C, De la Gandara B, Matallanas B, Reglero G, De Miguel E, June-July 2009.

Fitoterapia, *Carnosic Acid Inhibits the Growth of ER-Negative Human Breast Cancer Cells and Synergizes With Curcumin*, Einbond LS, Wu HA, Kashiwazaki R, He K, Roller M, Su T, Wang X, Goldsberry S, October 2012.

Food and Chemical Toxicology, *A Bioguided Identification of the Active Compounds that Contribute to the Antiproliferative/Cytotoxic Effects of Rosemary Extract on Colon Cancer Cells*, Borras-Linares I, Perez-Sanchez J, Barrajon-Catalan E, Arraez-Roman D, Cifuentes A, Micol V, Carretero AS, June 2015.

Food & Nutrition Research, *Skin Photoprotective and Antiaging Effects of a Combination of Rosemary (Rosmarinus officinalis) and Grapefruit (Citrus paradise) Polyphenols*, Nobile V, Michelotti A, Cestone E, Caturla N, Castillo J, Benavente-Garcia O, Perez-Sanchez A, Micol V, July 2016.

Food and Chemical Toxicology*, Potential of Long-Term Dietary Administration of Rosemary in Improving the Antioxidant Status of Rat Tissues Following Carbon Tetrachloride Intoxication*, Botsoglou N, Taitzoglou I, Zervos I, Botsoglou E, Tsantarliotou M, Chatzopoulou PS, March 2010.

Free Radical Biology & Medicine*, Photoprotective Potential of Lycopene, Beta-Carotene, Vitamin E, Vitamin C and Carnosic Acid in UVA-Irradiated Human Skin*, Offard EA, Gautier JC, Avanti O, Scaletta C, Runge F, Kramer K, Applegate LA, June 2002.

Holistic Nursing Practice*, The Effects of Lavender and Rosemary Essential Oils on Test-Taking Anxiety Among Graduate Nursing Students*, McCaffrey R, Thomas DJ, Kinzelman AO, March-April 2009.

Indian Journal of Experimental Biology*, Pharmacology of Rosemary (Rosmarinus officinalis Linn.) and its Therapeutic Potentials*, al Sereiti MR, Abu-Amer KM, Sen P, February 1999.

International Journal of Food Microbiology*, Antibacterial Activity of Selected Fatty Acids and Essential Oils Against Six Meat Spoilage Organisms*, Quattara B, Simard RE, Holley RA, Piette GJ, Begin A, July 1997.

International Journal of Food Sciences and Nutrition*, Anti-Oxidant, Anti-Glycant, and Inhibitory Activity Against Alpha-Amylase and Alpha-Glucosidase of Selected Spices and Culinary Herbs*, Cazzola R, Camerotto C, Cestaro B, March 2011.

International Journal of Neuroscience, *Aromas of Rosemary and Lavender Essential Oils Differentially Affect Cognition and Mood in Healthy Adults*, Moss M, Cook J, Wesmes K, Duckett P, January 2003.

International Journal of Tissue Reactions, *Induction of Heat Shock Protein Synthesis in Human Skin Fibroblasts in Response to Oxidative Stress: Regulation by a Natural Antioxidant from Rosemary Extract*, Calabrese V, Scapagnini G, Catalano C, Bates TE, Dinotta F, Micali G, Giuffrida Stella AM, 2001.

Investigative Opthalmology & Visual Science, *Protective Effect of Carnosic Acid, a Pro-Electrophilic Compound, in Models of Oxidative Stress and Light-Induced Retinal Degeneration*, Rezaie T, McKercher SR, Kosaka K, Seki M, Wheeler L, Viswanath V, Chun T, Joshi R, Valencia M, Sasaki S, Tozawa T, Satoh T, Lipton SA, November 2012.

Journal of Agricultural and Food Chemistry, *Bioactive Compounds from Culinary Herbs Inhibit a Molecular Target for Type 2 Diabetes Management, Dipeptidyl Peptidase IV*, Bower A, Hernandez L, Berhow M, Gonzalez de Mejia E, 2014.

Journal of Agricultural and Food Chemistry, *Protection of Dehydrated Chicken Meat by Natural Antioxidants as Evaluated by Electron Spin Resonance Spectrometry*, Nissin LR, Mansson L, Bertelsen G, Huynh-Ba T, Skibsted LH, November 2000.

Journal of Agricultural and Food Chemistry, *Rosemary (Rosmarinus officinalis L.) Extract Regulates Glucose and Lipid Metabolism by Activating AMPK and PPAR Pathways in HepG2 Cells*, Tu Z, Moss-Pierce T, Ford P, Jiang TA, March 2013.

Journal of Agricultural and Food Chemistry, *Testing and Enhancing the In Vitro Bioaccessibility and Bioavailability of Rosmarinus officinalis Extracts With a High Level of Antioxidant Abietanes*, Soler-Rivas C, Marin FR, Santoyo S, Garcia-Risco MR, Senorans FJ, Relero G, January 2010.

Journal of Alternative and Complementary Medicine, *Effect of the Herbal Combination Canephron N on Diabetic Nephropathy in Patients with Diabetes Mellitus: Results of a Comparative Cohort Study*, Martynyuk L, Martynyuk L, Ruzhitska O, Martynyuk O, June 2014.

Journal of Animal Science and Biotechnology, *Dietary Supplementation of Rosmarinus officinalis L. Leaves in Sheep Affects the Abundance of Rumen Methanogens and other Microbial Populations*, Cobellis G, Yu Z, Acuti G, Trabalza-Marinucci M, April 2016.

Journal of Ethnopharmacology, *Healing Potential of Rosmarinus officinalis L. on Full-Thickness Excision Cutaneous Wounds in Alloxan-Induced-Diabetic BALB/c Mice*, Abu-Al-Basal MA, September 2010.

Journal of Ethnopharmacology, *In Vivo Assessment of Antidiabetic and Antioxidant Activities of Rosemary (Rosmarinus officinalis) in Alloxan-Diabetic Rabbits*, Bakirel T, Bakirel U, Keles OU, Ulgen SG, Yardibi H, February 2008.

Journal of Medicinal Food, *Short-term Study on the Effects of Rosemary on Cognitive Function in an Elderly Population*, Pengelly A, Snow J, Mills SY, Scholey A, Wesnes K, Butler LR, August 2011.

Journal of Photochemistry and Photobiology:B, *Protective Effects of Citrus and Rosemary Extracts on UV-Induced Damage in Skin Cell Model and Human Volunteers*, Perez-Sanchez A, Barrajon-Catalan E, Caturla N, Castillo J, Benavente-Garcia O, Alcaraz M, Micol V, July 2014.

Journal of Physiology and Biochemistry, *Hypoglycemic and Hepatoprotective Activity of Rosmarinus officinalis Extract in Diabetic Rats*, Ramadan KS, Khalil OA, Danial EN, Alnahdi HS, Ayaz NO, December 2013.

Lamb, The Good Cook: Techniques & Recipes Series, Editors of Time-Life, 1981.

LaRousse Gastronomique: The New American Edition of the World's Greatest Culinary Encyclopedia, Jenifer Harvey Lang, Editor, Crown Publishers, 1988.

Meat Science, *The Oxidative Activity of Plant Extracts in Cooked Pork Patties as Evaluated by Descriptive Sensory Profiling and Chemical Analysis*, Nissen LR, Byrne DV. Bertelsen G, Skibsted LH, November 2004.

Medical Journal of The Islamic Republic of Iran, *The Effect of Rosemary Extract on Spatial Memory, Learning and Antioxidant Enzymes Activities in the Hippocampus of Middle-Aged Rats*, Rasoolijazi H, Mehdizadeh M, Soleimani M, Nikbakhte F, Eslami Farsani M, Ababzadeh S, March 2015.

Molecular Vision, *Prevention of Retinal Light Damage by Zinc Oxide Combined With Rosemary Extract*, Organisciak DT, Darrow RM, Rapp CM, Smuts JP, Armstrong DW, Lang JC, June 2013.

Molecules, *Rosmarinic Acid, A Rosemary Extract Polyphenol, Increases Skeletal Muscle Cell Glucose Uptake and Activates AMPK*, Vlavcheski F, Naimi M, Hudlicky T, Tsiani E, October 2017.

Molecules, *The Potential Of Use Basil and Rosemary Essential Oils as Effective Antibacterial Agents*, Sienkiewicz M, Lysakowska M, Pastuszka M, Bienias W, Kowalczyk E, August 2013.

Nauyn-Schmiedeberg's Archives of Pharmacology, *Rosemary (Rosemarinus officinalis) as a Potential Therapeutic Plant in Metabolic Syndrome: A Review*, Hassani FV, Shirani K, Hosseinzadeh H, September 2016.

Neuroscience Letters, *Rosemary Extract Improves Cognitive Deficits In A Rats Model of Repetitive Mild Traumatic Brain Injury Associated With Reduction of Astrocytosis and Neuronal Degeneration in Hippocampus*, Song H, Xu L, Zhang R, Cao Z, Zhang H, Yang L, Guo Z, Qu Y, Yu J, May 2016.

Nutrients, *Anticancer Effects of Rosemary (Rosmarinus officinalis L.) Extract and Rosemary Extract Polyphenols*, Moore J, Yousef M, Tsiani E, November 2016.

Nutrition and Cancer, *Carnosic Acid Inhibits Proliferation and Augments Differentiation of Human Leukemic Cells Induced by 1,25-dihydroxyvitamin D3 and Retinoic Acid*, Steiner M, Priel I, Giat J, Levy J, Sharoni Y, Danilenko M, 2001.

Nutrition and Cancer, *Rosemary (Rosmarinus officinalis L.) Extract as a Potential Complementary Agent in Anticancer Therapy*, Gonzalez-Vallinas M, Reglero G, Ramirez de Molina A, October 2015.

Nutrition Industry Executive, *Field-to-Fork Organic Rosemary Solutions From Frutarom*, July-August 2017.

Pathophysiology, *Rosemary (Rosemarinus officinalis) Essential Oil Components Exhibit Anti-Hyperglycemic, Anti-Hyperlipidemic and Antioxidant Effects in Experimental Diabetes*, Selmi S, Rtibi K, Grami D, Sebai H, Marzouki L, September 2017.

Pharmaceutical Biology, *Transdermal Absorption Enhancing Effect of the Essential Oil of Rosmarinus officinalis on Percutaneous Absorption of Na Diclofenac From Topical Gel*, Akbari J, Saeedi M, Farzin D, Morteza-Semnani K, Esmaili Z, April, 2015.

Pharmaceutics, *Rosemary Essential Oil-Loaded Lipid Nanoparticles: In Vivo Topical Activity From Gel Vehicles*, Montenegro L, Pasquinucci L, Zappala A, Chiechio S, Turnaturi R, Parenti C, October 2017.

Photochemistry and Photobiology, *Modulation of Photochemical Damage in Normal and Malignant Cells by Naturally Occurring Compounds*, Lee YH, Kumar NC, Glickman RD, November-December 2012.

Phytomedicine, *Antiproliferation Effect of Rosemary (Rosmarinus officinalis) on Human Ovarian Cancer Cells In Vitro*, Taj J, Cheung S, Wu M, Hasman D, March 2012.

Phytotherapy Research, *Effect of Rosmarinus officinalis in Modulating 7,12-dimethylbenz(a)anthracene Induced Skin Tumorigenesis in Mice*, Sancheti G, Goyal PK, November 2006.

Phytotherapy Research, *Phenolic Diterpenes from Rosemary Suppress cAMP Responsiveness of Gluconeogenic Gene Promoters*, Yun YS, Noda S, Shigemori G, Kuriyama R, Umemura M, Takahashi Y, Inoue H, June, 2013.

Plant Foods for Human Nutrition, *Carotenoid Content of Commonly Consumed Herbs and Assessment of their Bioaccessibility Using an In Vitro Digestion Model*, Daly T, Jiwan MA, O'Brien, NM, Aherne SA, June 2010.

Plant Foods for Human Nutrition, *Inhibitory Effects of Rosemary Extracts, Carnosic Acid and Rosmarinic Acid on the Growth of Various Human Cancer Cell Lines*, Yesil-Celiktas O, Sevimli C, Bedir E, Vardar-Sukan F, June,2010.

PLOS One Augophagy Research, *Anti-Proliferative Effect of Rosmarinus officinalis L. Extract on Human Melanoma A375 Cells*, Cattaneo L, Cicconi R, Mignogna G, Giorgi A, Mattei M, Graziani G, Ferracane R, Grosso A, Aducci P, Schinina ME, Marra M, July 2015.

PLOS One Autophagy Research, *Expression of MicroRNA-15b and the Glycosyltransferase GCNT3 Correlates With Antitumor Efficacy of Rosemary Diterpenes in Colon and Pancreatic Cancer*, Gonzalez-Vallinas M, Molina S, Vicente G, Zarza V, Martin-Hernandez R, Garcia-Risco, MR, Fornari T, Reglero G, Ramirez de Molina A, June 2014.

PLOS One Autophagy Research, *Rosemary (Rosmarinus officinalis) Extract Modulates CHOP/GADD153 to Promote Androgen Receptor Degradation and Decreases Xenograft Tumor Growth*, Petiwala SM, Berhe S, Li G, Puthenveetil AG, Rahman O, Nonn L, Johnson JJ, March 2014.

PLOS One Autophagy Research, *Rosemary Supplementation (Rosemarinus officinallis L.) Attenuates Cardiac Remodeling After Myocardial Infarction In Rats,*

Murino Rafacho BP, Portugal Dos Santos P, Goncalves AF, Fernandes AAH, Okoshi K, Chiuso-Minicucci F, Azevedo PS, Mamede Zornoff LA, Minicucci MF, Wang XD, Rupp de Paiva SA, May 2017.

Poultry Science, *Influence of Two Plant Extracts on Broilers Performance, Digestibility, and Digestive Organ Size*, Hernandez F, Madrid J, Garcia V, Orengo J, Megias MD, February 2004.

Poultry Science, *Oxidative Stability of the Meat of Broilers Supplemented with Rosemary Leaves, Rosehip Fruits, Chokeberry Pomace, and Entire Nettle, and Effects on Performance and Meat Quality*, Loetscher Y, Kreuzer M, Messikommer RE, November 2013.

Poultry Science, *The Effect of Herbs and Their Associated Essential Oils on Performance, Dietary Digestibility and Gut Microflora in Chickens From 7 to 28 Days of Age*, Cross DE, McDevitt RM, Hillman K, Acamovic T, August 2007.

Professional's Handbook of Complementary & Alternative Medicines, Fetrow, Charles W., PharmD; Avila, Juan R, PharmD, Springhouse, Inc., 1999.

Proven Herbal Blends: A Rational Approach to Prevention and Remedy, Mowrey, Daniel B., Keats Publishing, 1986.

Psychiatry Research, *Smelling Lavender and Rosemary Increases Free Radical Scavenging Activity and Decreases Cortisol Level in Saliva*, Atsumi T, Tonosaki K, February 2007.

Scientia Pharmaceutica, *Effects of Inhaled Rosemary Oil on Subjective Feelings and Activities of the Nervous System*, Sayorway VV, Ruangrugsi N, Piriyapunyporn T, Hongratanaworakit T, Kotchabhakdi N, Siripornpanich V, April-June, 2013.

SKINmed, *Rosemary Oil Vs Minoxidil 2% for the Treatment of Androgenetic Alopecia: A Randomized Comparative Trial*, Pahahi Y, Tahizadeh M, Marzony ET, Sahebkar A, January-February 2015.

St. Martin de Porres: Apostle of Charity, 1942, Cavallini, Guiliana.

The Herb Book, Arabella Boxer & Phillipa Back, 1988. (Gallery Books).

Acknowledgements

Many thanks to Kathryn E. King, who aided me with every aspect of this book.

About The Author

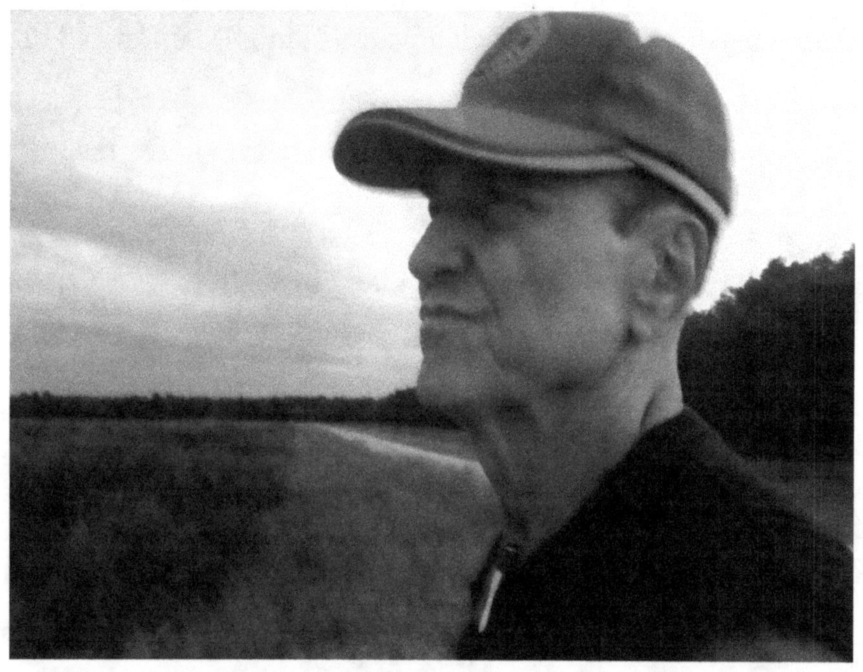

Dr. Charles S. Brocato is a scientist and author who has written extensively in the fields of surviving chemical and biological warfare and nuclear warfare. He is also a longtime martial arts instructor, specializing in *how to stay alive*. He is also a nutritionist and a counselor in the field of nutrition.

He holds degrees in biology and mathematics with advanced studies in the areas of biochemistry and microbiology, and a Ph.D. in theology. He is also an award-winning French chef.

Two of his previous books are available on Amazon in print form: *The Two-Fold Chastisement: Visions of the Coming Earth Changes*, and *Chemical/Biological WarFare: How You Can Survive.*

This book is the result of his studies in nutrition and French cooking, combined with his interest in the way St. Martin de Porres used rosemary to such advantage in 17th-century Peru.